HEALING FLOWERS A-Z

By
DIANE STEIN

LOTUS
PRESS

P.O. Box 325
Twin Lakes, WI 53181 USA

DISCLAIMER

Healing and medicine are two very different fields, and the law requires a disclaimer. The information of this book is metaphysical rather than medical and does not constitute medical advice. In case of illness, consult the professional of your choice.

Lotus Press
P.O. Box 325
Twin Lakes, WI 53181 USA
800-824-6396 (toll free order phone)
262-889-8561 (office phone)
262-889-2461 (office fax)
www.lotuspress.com (website)
lotuspress@lotuspress.com (email)

ISBN: 978-0-9406-7698-5

Library of Congress Control Number: 2011938217

Contents

ILLUSTRATIONS

INTRODUCTION:

Healing With Flowers

Flowers are beautiful, we all know that. When most people think of the beauty of the Earth, flowers are almost the first thing in mind. Flowers are also healers. Plants were the first medicines, using herbs (prepared and ingested plant parts including flowers) to fight dis-ease, calm the mind and balance the body. They have been known to every continent and culture since prehistory. In 1933, Dr. Edward Bach published his pamphlet <u>The Twelve Healers and Other Remedies</u> in England and the flowers of plants became a new (or possibly rediscovered) focus for healing. Where herbs require ingestion of plant parts (leaves, stems, roots or flowers), healing flowers use an energy imprint of the flower life force.

Dr. Bach developed a system for preparing and using thirty-eight flowers (plus the Rescue Remedy combination). He thoroughly researched what each flower would do as a healing energy. He made his flower essences, as they were called, in the way that homeopathic remedies are still made. Later investigators of flower healing developed simpler preparation methods and explored different flowers, building upon Dr. Bach's work. They developed easier ways to make essences and explored what various flowers could do as healing tools. I have been one of those investigators for the last fifteen years.

While herbs work upon the function of the physical body, flower essences are much more subtle. A flower essence is an imprint of a flower, not the flower itself—unlike with herbs, no plant or plant material is ever ingested in a flower essence. As Dr. Bach knew, they are closer to homeopathic remedies, which are also energy imprints, in how they work. Flower essence effects are less physiological and work more upon the energy of the spirit than of the body. While an herb may be used to sedate, for example, a flower essence might be used to promote peace of mind. While an herb might be used to relieve a dis-ease, a flower essence might be used with many dis-eases to help the sufferer endure patiently or to support the body's healing strength during other treatment.

Dr. Bach investigated thirty-eight flowers that grew in his English neighborhood. It has long been known by herbalists that the most potent healing herbs are those that grow where one lives. The flowers that bloom in Florida are quite different from those that bloom in England, and likewise the flowers that will grow in California or Nebraska or Arizona or Russia. There are many thousands of flowering plants, all with their own potential as energetic healers. There is very good reason to look to the flowers of home for healing, wherever home may be. This opens up the possibilities that Dr. Bach began to discover, and makes the possibilities of flower essences for healing virtually limitless.

Gemstones are also part of the beauty of the Earth and are powerful energies for healing. (When you thought of the beauty of the Earth, if you didn't think of flowers first, you thought of gemstones!) I have worked so long with gemstones as healers that I automatically include them in whatever energetic healing I may do. When I began to study the flowers around me and make them into essences, it was natural to add gemstones to the flowers in making my essences. When I knew a flower would help to bring about peace of mind, it was automatic to think "like Rose Quartz does" or "this flower feels like Celestite". As I moved more into studying essences I began combining my flowers with compatible gemstones. The resulting essences were much more powerful and the gemstones could be used to more fully focus the use of the essence.

This book contains the channeled uses for 350 flowers. Each flower is listed with its Latin name for identification, its color, and which chakra the essence is most focused upon for healing. Chakras are the energy centers of the nonphysical bodies and will be discussed more below. With each flower entry is also listed a group of possible gemstones to include in making the essence, to enhance and increase its healing abilities. The flower will do what is described, whether gemstones are added to the essence or not, but adding one or more of the listed gemstones with greatly strengthen it.

Several gemstones are listed with each flower entry, but only one or two are needed in the essence you will make of that flower. Pick the gemstone (or gemstones) that you are drawn to in the list or the ones from the list that are available. Each list of gemstones includes Danburite, which can be used with other stones to greatly enhance and balance any flower essence. In addition to the other stones you choose, including Danburite will magnify and focus any essence and is much recommended for all of them. Also, every essence lists either Clear Quartz Crystal or Herkimer Diamond. If you have these stones, add one or the other to the gemstones in the essences you make. They also magnify and focus the plant energy, and help to transfer the flower's life force imprint into the essences.

Flower essences are something anyone can easily learn to make, and this book is about making your own. Dr. Bach's work is well-known and there is no need to duplicate it here. These essences are made in your own garden from the flowers that grow there. The tools needed are available in most kitchens, but if you choose to preserve your essences to keep longer than the day they are made, you will need to have bottles for them—larger bottles for the Mother Tinctures (pint or quart), less large bottles for the preparation dilution (about 4 oz.), and small dropper bottles (1/2 or 1 oz.) for the last dilution and dosage use. These bottles need to be dark colored glass to protect the essences from light once they are made; they can usually be purchased from pharmacies.

In addition to storage bottles, you will need a clear glass bowl (stainless steel will work, but not plastic), and pure water—spring or filtered water, rather than tap water. Essences are mostly made in sunlight on a sunny day, though nightblooming flowers are best made at night under a Full Moon. You need the flower in bloom—pick it only when it will go immediately into essence using a food-clean scissor to cut it from the plant. You also need the gemstones to be included, and these should be energetically cleansed in sea salt for at least several hours before they are rinsed off and put into the essence bowl.

To make your essence, fill the clear glass bowl with spring water. Place in it the gemstones you have chosen, and then pick (cut with clean scissors) the flowers to go into the bowl. Remove the stems and leaves. Only the blossom itself is used, and used whole (do not cut up the flower or petals, use the whole intact flower). You need two or three blossoms at least, or enough floating flowers to lightly cover the surface of the water. If a flower is very large, or only one flower is blooming, one will do. Pick the most beautiful and perfectly formed of the flowers available, touch them as little as possible, and place them in the bowl of water. If you know Reiki, place a Reiki attunement or the Cho-Ku-Rei symbol over it. Leave the bowl in the sun (or under the moonlight) for about four hours.

After four hours, remove the flowers (I like to give them back to the Earth) and bring the bowl indoors—this is your Mother

Tincture. If you are going to use the essence once and throw the rest away, place two drops of the water (now your Mother Tincture flower essence) in a glass of spring water and drink it. The water will keep only through the day if no preservative is added. If it begins to develop an odor or a film, throw it away.

If you wish to keep your essence for later use, you must bottle and preserve it. To do this, put about an inch of brandy or vodka in a brown glass quart bottle (or half that in a pint brown glass bottle) and fill the rest with the Mother Tincture. To avoid alchohol you can also use white vinegar or a strong tea of the herb red shiso (perilla) as the preservative. The bottle needs to have a tight screw-on cap to close it with.

The preserved Mother Tincture is very potent and has to be diluted. Unpreserved, you used two drops in a water glass (16 oz.) of pure water. Preserved, take a 4 oz. brown glass bottle, put a quarter inch of brandy (or vodka, vinegar or perilla) in it, eight drops of the Mother Tincture, and add pure water to fill. Close the bottle and shake it a few times to mix the ingredients. This is your preparation bottle, which you will dilute one more time.

Next, take your half ounce or one ounce brown glass dropper bottle. Put about a teaspoonful of preservative in the one ounce bottle (half that in the half ounce bottle), add four drops of essence from the preparation bottle, and fill to half an inch from the top with pure water. This is your dosage bottle. From this bottle, take two to four drops of the essence three or four times a day, straight from the dropper. You can also place the drops in a glass of water, in tea (especially herbal tea) or in juice. If you know Reiki, you can repeat the attunement or Cho-Ku-Rei with each step in bottling.

Two cautions here. First, flowers used in making essences should not be eaten. An essence is an energy imprint of the flower, not the flower itself. No flower should be eaten unless you know it to be an edible plant. Many flowers are toxic or poisonous; the essence will not be. Second, flower essences are not fragrances—those are essential oils. Your essence will smell slightly of the flower if you use it fresh, slightly of the preservative if you have bottled it. Flower essences are taken by mouth, two to four drops of the dosage bottle dilution taken straight or in other liquid. Essential oils are never to be taken internally unless under the direction of an aromatherapy expert; they are for external use only and even a drop or two can be highly toxic. Many people confuse flower essences with essential oils—we are making and using flower essences in this book.

The uses for the flowers in this book have been channeled, which means that they are comprised of information given to me by Light Be-ings—healers and helpers who are not in body. Such helpers can include spirit guides, angels, other-planetary healers and teachers, one's Higher Self, or even a Goddess. Because the information source is so unique—and I highly trust it—the flower definitions in this book may not match others' definitions for the same flower. Part of this is because every expert, including those who are not in body, has their own definitions of what a flower (or herb, or gemstone) will do. Part of this is also because of the unique addition of gemstones to the essence mix. The stones enhance the essences and focus their uses, thereby increasing their ability to help and heal. I will stand by my channeled essence definitions but agree that others' differing meanings may also be as accurate.

An interesting consideration in the uses of flowers for healing is the Victorian Language of Flowers. It was almost an art in the England of Queen Victoria to put a clear message or meaning to the use of a flower sent in a bouquet to a friend or love interest. While these were not healing meanings, they could sometimes be revealing of what energy the flower carried. Roses symbolized love, of course. But to offer a bouquet of tulips was to make a declaration of one's love for the receiver of the bouquet. Iris meant hope and wisdom, sunflowers were aspiration and longevity, asters were patience, and lily of the valley the return of happiness. A few of these meanings are noted in this book, but because of lack of space there are only a few. If you wish to pursue this information, which is also called floriography, do an online search for the meaning of flowers. There is also a small anonymous book called The Language of Flowers that has remained continuously in print since 1913 and lists hundreds of flower language meanings.

The flower essences in this book often have use for healing damage to the nonphysical energy bodies and chakras. The human energy field (aura) extends through a great many levels, called energy bodies. Most people in metaphysics are aware of the physical, emotional, mental and spiritual bodies. These are the basics, and are the levels closest to the physical body we know. They are only a small beginning of the complexies of human or animal energy, however. For this book and use of flower essences, the four bodies will be mentioned frequently. Each of these four bodies also has a higher "octave" that some essences are powerful enough to heal.

The higher level of the physical body is the etheric body or etheric double; this is the nonphysical energy duplicate of the physical body. Next, the emotional body's higher octave is the astral body, and the astral twin is what we usually call our inner child. The mental body has a higher level also, called the mind grid. The mind grid is almost an energetic computer that contains the blueprint of our individual creation. This is the place that is reprogrammed when karma is released. The higher octave of the spiritual body has two parts to it, the galactic body and the causal body, but causal body or causal level can be used to refer to both parts.

While most people are aware of the kundalini chakras, they are the chakras for the physical-etheric body only. Each body has its own chakra system. Occasionally, flower essences described in this book reach higher than the etheric body and provide healing for higher bodies and their chakras. This usually means the emotional-astral body, and the chakras for this level are called the hara line or hara chakras. A discussion of the kundalini and hara line chakras is at the end of this introduction, placed there for easy referal. Essences occasionally reach the mental body-mind grid level, and rarely the causal body level for healing. The aura is the energy field or envelop that surrounds each octave of energy bodies. For a full discussion of energy anatomy and the bodies and chakras see my book <u>Essential Energy Balancing</u> (The Crossing Press, 2000).

There are a few other terms that come up in the flower essence entries that may be unfamiliar. Karma is one such subject. Karma is unhealed trauma from past lifetimes (or from this life) that causes ongoing or repeated suffering until the original situation is released (cleared or healed). Karmic release is a great gift to us now, and some flower essences help in the work of releasing karma. Again, if this is a subject that interests you, see <u>Essential Energy Balancing</u>.

Another frequent term is "heart scars" (which are also karmic). A heart scar is metaphorically what the words say—a scar on the emotional heart, a concentration of emotional pain. This is from the great hurts, disappointments, losses, griefs and traumas in one's life—the great incidents of heartbreak that everyone experiences. When a heart scar is released, however, it may be a very unpleasant experience—it comes with a reliving of the trauma and possibly physical pain. But when the release is over, a feeling of great relief remains, followed by a great weight lifted from one's life and a lighter heart. Some flowers can be used to release these scars gently and they accomplish a profound healing.

In another definition, chakra complexes are the chakras through all levels and bodies—for example the heart complex is the heart chakra on all the (108) body levels. The levels are intertwined, and healing a chakra complex is major core soul healing.

Ascension or enlightenment is also a subject that appears frequently in the flower essence meanings. Enlightenment is a Buddhist term that means that the person will complete their requirement to reincarnate with this life time. It means that at their death they have resolved all of their karma, their suffering and their need to learn how to avoid suffering, and therefore they no longer are required to return to the physical body. Some who complete enlightenment, however, choose to reincarnate again for the purpose of helping others to attain enlightenment. These are the bodhisattvas, Kwan Yin being the best known example. However, a great many ordinary people are bodisattvas, know it or not, here on Earth to help and to heal. We have incarnated (lived life times in a physical body) a great many times; the body may change but the soul is eternal.

Ascension is basically enlightenment but with a difference. In this case, when the person completes the release of all their karma to a particular level, something different happens. Instead of having no need to return to Earth for another incarnation after one's death, the enlightenment is completed on Earth now. When the karmic debt is resolved, the person's soul is brought into their body. They remain very much alive and in this life time continue their work on Earth. As an ascended Be-ing, they have a responsibility to help others and to help in the healing of the planet. They may bring in a Goddess (or God if male) to work through them. Though they have completed their incarnational requirements, they now use that ascension energy to help others. They become bodhisattvas, with a job to do for this life time as an ascended enlightened Be-ing. This is a much to be desired goal of spirituality, this high level service to the Light, though it is not for everyone. Again, if you are interested in achieving this, see my series of Essential Energy Balancing books.

Since each flower essence is matched to a kundalini or hara line chakra, some brief information on the chakras is in order here. The kundalini chakras are the series of seven energy centers that run down the center front of the body, and most people involved with metaphysics and healing are familiar with them. These chakras are located on the etheric body level, the energy level closest to the physical body. Chakras are receptors that bring in energies from the Earth below and the Light above. How well we are able to process these energies determines our state of physical health. Each chakra works to regulate a different aspect of physical life, including our basic emotions and mental states.

Each chakra has a corresponding color (the alternate colors I often use are mostly for the hara line described below, except for the heart chakra where two colors are generally accepted). The colors of the flowers and gemstones are used in each essence to match the chakra colors. For example, if the heart chakra's color correspondences are green and pink, pink flowers would correspond to the heart chakra and gemstones added to the essence are usually pink. Sometimes a white flower uses green or pink gemstones to comprise a heart chakra essence. These flower and gemstone colors support healing for the heart physically and/or emotionally. They may even provide healing for the entire heart complex. The definitions of which flowers or gemstones match each chakra, beyond the color correpondences, are not rigid.

Beginning with the kundalini chakras, the first chakra is the **Root Chakra**, located at the genitals, the flower color is red and the gemstones are red or black. (There are only a very few black flowers.) The root is the seat of the life force, survival and one's core identity, as well as the place of grounding, centering, and reducing anger. There are many red flowers, but only a few red gemstones.

Next is the **Belly Chakra**, located below the navel, whose corresponding color is orange. The belly is the seat of sexuality, birth, menstruation, sensuality, fertility, sexual relationships, desire (more than sexual desire), passion of all types, and some forms of creativity. Pictures and visions of old hurts and traumas may be stored in the belly chakra until they are resolved and released. The flowers and added gemstones for this chakra are orange or yellow-orange in color.

The **Solar Plexus** follows, located at the waist between the lowest pair of ribs, and associated with the color yellow. It is the place of perceptual feeling, assimilation of psychic impressions, digestion, physical energy distribution, and mental energy, intellect and the mind. Yellow and golden yellow flowers and gemstones are used for this chakra, like sunflowers or yellow petaled daisies. Golden gemstones are added, like Topaz or Yellow Jade.

Next, the **Heart Chakra** is located beneath the breastbone at the center of the chest. Heart chakra healing involves the emotions, the physical heart, compassion for oneself and others, a postive self-image, and a sense of connectedness—understanding the oneness of all life. The colors are green or pink. There are a very few green flowers, however, so heart chakra flowers are primarily pink ones. They are usually supported by pink gemstones like Rose Quartz.

The **Throat Chakra**, at the lower front of the throat, with its light blue color, brings healing to the physical throat, as well as healing and support for speech, singing, acting, writing, creativity, speaking one's truth, and speaking one's needs. Its primary attributes are expression, particularly expression of personal truth. There are a limited number of blue flowers, like blue sage, and their uses always revolve around truth and speaking out. Some light blue gemstones include Celestite or Blue Chalcedony.

The **Third Eye Chakra**, which is above and between the eyes, corresponds to dark blue or indigo. This chakra heals and supports vision, psychic vision, clairvoyance, perceptions of psychic and physical reality, whole body purification, and energy repair and re-programming. Indigo flowers and gemstones for the third eye bring about spiritual transformations, but they may not work gently.

The **Crown Chakra**, located just behind the top of the head, is the spriituality center of the physical-etheric body levels. It brings in energy and information from the Light above, and then provides all our impressions of what is beyond life—beyond our physical consciousness. The color in flowers and gemstones both is purple (violet, lavender) or white. Think of lilac flowers and the gemstone Amethyst. There are not a great many purple flowers, and even fewer purple gemstones.

The thirteen hara line chakras are on the emotional-astral energy body, a step further away from the physical, beyond the etheric body and kundalini system. These chakras are less known but incrasingly important in healing, since all healing these days involves emotional healing. From the top down, the chakras and colors of the hara line follow.

The **Transpersonal Point** is located beyond the crown, being a higher level of it, above the physical body. This point connects us with our core soul and with all energy components beyond the physical for higher level spirituality. Its color is clear, and white flowers with white or clear gemstones are usually used for this center.

The next chakras are a pair behind each eye called **Vision Chakras**, which enable one to do laser healing with the eyes. They are also used for all types of psychic vision and psychic seeing. The color for these centers is silver or grey. Since this is rarely a flower color (and not much less rarely a gemstone color), there are only a few flower essences that target the vision chakras.

Below that, at the back of the head, where the skull meets the top of the neck, is the **Casual Body Chakra**. This is the seat of receiving spiritual information and manifesting it into useful and understandable form. It includes channeling, clairaudience (psychic hearing), automatic writing, and communication from spirit guides and other Light Be-ings. The color for this chakra when activated is crimson or red-violet. Before opening, this chakra's color is silver-blue. There are a number of crimson or red-violet flowers to represent this chakra and a few silver-blue ones, but a limited number of either color gemstones. Pink Tourmaline is a red-violet stone, and Blue Kyanite a silver-blue one.

Next is the **Thymus Chakra**, the high heart that is the heart center of the hara line. This center is located about two inches above the physical breast bone and it hurts when you press it. Its uses are to protect the physical heart and immune systems, heal grief, and protect the emotions. It is also a bridge between the heart and throat chakras—feeling and expression of feeling. This chakra's color is turquoise or aqua—not a common flower color, but there are a number of corresponding gemstones.

The **Diaphragm Chakra**, lime green or yellow green, is the hara line equivalent of the solar plexus. This is the center for emotional cleansing and detoxification of emotions, and it is not a comfortable center to work with. There are a very few green flowers (hothouse bred) and a few that are yellow-green; Green Goddess Amaryllis comes to mind. Green Amber or Green Kunzite (Hiddenite) are gemstone examples for this center.

The **Hara Chakra** is located between the kundalini root and the belly chakra, which are on the energy level below it. It is the seat of one's life purpose and provides the stability to achieve and manifest it. It is the body's central balance point, and its colors are golden, gold-brown, orange-brown or even dark red. There are a number of flowers for this chakra, like yellow loosetrife; in gemstones Amber is primary and there are a number of other golden stones.

The hara line **Perineum Chakra** is equivalaent to the kundalini root, located between the genitals and the anal opening. It is the first chakra of the grounding system and is about bringing one's life purpose into physical form. Its color is maroon—like a dark red peony flower, or a Ruby gemstone.

A pair of chakras called **Movement Chakras** is located at the backs of the knees. Their color is dark green or tan, and they aid forward movement on one's path. There are a rare few of tan flowers, and the primary gemstone is dark green Moldavite or any of the brown Jaspers. These chakras are also part of the grounding system.

The **Grounding Chakras** are located on the bottoms of both feet. Their color is brown, and they represent our connection to the physical world. A very few flowers (brown or not) heal these chakras, and all the brown Jasper gemstones operate here.

Below the feet, beyond the physical body, is the EARTH CHAKRA or Earth Star which connects us to and with the planet itself. This chakra's color is black—there are a very few black or red-black flowers that work for this chakra, among them the black calla lily called Captain Palermo. Many black gemstones, however, help with this vital connecting, without which we are no longer alive. Black Tourmaline is a good gemstone for this energy center.

As I mentioned previously the correspondence of flowers to specific chakra colors is not rigid, less rigid than the gemstones. Where the flower color does not seem to correspond, I can only speculate that the plant energy corresponds even if its color seems questionable. Channeled information works like that sometimes—I can only go with it, and ask you to do so too. Illustrations of the kundalini and hara line chakras follow.

Flowers are beautiful and fascinating energies to work with, as are gemstones. Together they are powerful and have great consequence to help and heal. I hope that the information in this book will make you curious enough to start making your own flower essences. They are important healers at a time when the Earth and all who live here badly need their healing.

ILLUSTRATION 1.
THE KUNDALINI CHAKRAS

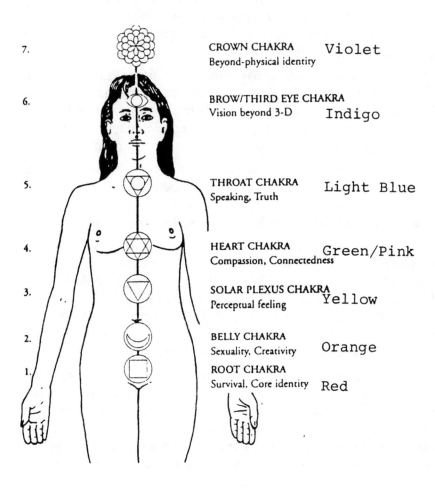

7.   **CROWN CHAKRA**   Violet
            Beyond-physical identity

6.   **BROW/THIRD EYE CHAKRA**
            Vision beyond 3-D   Indigo

5.   **THROAT CHAKRA**   Light Blue
            Speaking, Truth

4.   **HEART CHAKRA**   Green/Pink
            Compassion, Connectedness

3.   **SOLAR PLEXUS CHAKRA**   Yellow
            Perceptual feeling

2.   **BELLY CHAKRA**
            Sexuality, Creativity   Orange

1.   **ROOT CHAKRA**
            Survival, Core identity   Red

ILLUSTRATION 2.
THE HARA LINE CHAKRAS

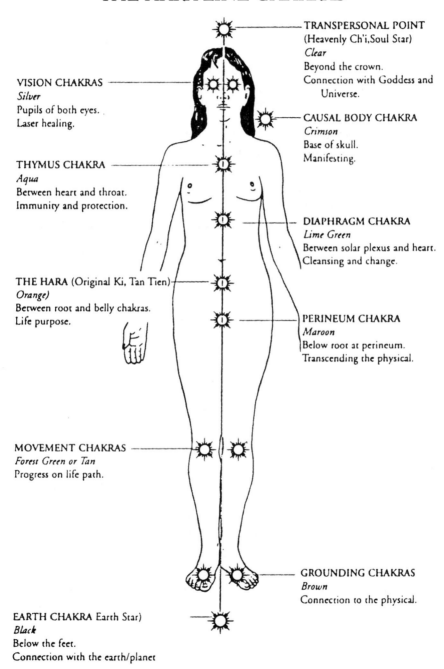

TRANSPERSONAL POINT
(Heavenly Ch'i, Soul Star)
Clear
Beyond the crown.
Connection with Goddess and
Universe.

VISION CHAKRAS
Silver
Pupils of both eyes.
Laser healing.

CAUSAL BODY CHAKRA
Crimson
Base of skull.
Manifesting.

THYMUS CHAKRA
Aqua
Between heart and throat.
Immunity and protection.

DIAPHRAGM CHAKRA
Lime Green
Between solar plexus and heart.
Cleansing and change.

THE HARA (Original Ki, Tan Tien)
Orange)
Between root and belly chakras.
Life purpose.

PERINEUM CHAKRA
Maroon
Below root at perineum.
Transcending the physical.

MOVEMENT CHAKRAS
Forest Green or Tan
Progress on life path.

GROUNDING CHAKRAS
Brown
Connection to the physical.

EARTH CHAKRA Earth Star)
Black
Below the feet.
Connection with the earth/planet

HEALING FLOWERS A-Z

AFRICAN TULIP TREE
(Spathodea campanulata)
(Perineum) Red

> **Add Gemstones:** Garnet, Black Velvet Tourmaline, Obsidian, Black Sapphire, Black Star Sapphire, Smoky Quartz, Onyx, Black Coral, Clear Quartz Crystal, Danburite
>
> Resolves karmic issues of dying and incarnating, all karma regarding death and rebirth; clears negative entities and attachments from the chakras, aura and energy bodies; heals the aura of negativity and evil interference, releases possessions, passes-over spirits stuck on Earth; releases negative karmic patterns, change negative thinking to positive; releases anger and resentment

AKEBIA VINE
(Akebia quinata)

(Crown) Purple

> **Add Gemstones:** Violet Tourmaline, Pink Tourmaline, Purple Kunzite, Sugilite, Alexandrite, Purple Sapphire, Phenacite, Herkimer Diamond, Danburite
>
> Provides and increases contact with one's beyond-physical inner self and soul, promotes increased contact with one's energy selves (Higher Self, Essence Self, Goddess Self) and Goddess; increases awareness of oneself as a spiritual Be-ing; clears, heals and activates the spiritual and causal (higher level spiritual) bodies, facilitates core soul healing, facilitates DNA repair; increases access and communication with spirit guides and angels, promotes receiving and understanding spiritual information, aids channeling and intuition; aids all ascension and enlightenment processes, promotes all spirituality, purifies

ALLAMANDA
(Allamanda cathartica)

(Grounding) Brown

Add Gemstones: Pietersite, Brown Jasper, Boulder Opal, Shiva Lingam, Smoky Quartz, Tiger Eye, Astrophyllite, Elestial Quartz, Clear Quartz Crystal, Danburite

For stabile rootedness into the earth plane, provides grounding and centering, helps keep one connected to the planet, connects the grounding cord to the planet core; promotes increased strength in walking one's life path, provides certainty of life purpose; protects and repairs the aura, heals the grounding system and its energy components, keeps astral travelers safe while out of body; promotes Earth awareness; inspires a life of balance and harmony, stability and steadiness, innate responsibility. Also called Chocolate Allamanda.

ALLAMANDA
(Allamanda cathartica)

(Hara) Peach

Add Gemstones: Peach Aventurine, Peach Moonstone, Peach Calcite, Mexican Opal, Jelly Opal, Peach Sunstone, Feldspar, Herkimer Diamond, Danburite

Promotes deep core soul healing; clears, heals and opens several of the higher aura bodies and their chakra systems (especially the etheric and emotional bodies); heals damage and tears in the etheric and emotional body auras, heals the astral body, repairs electrical malfunctions in the aura and auric field on all levels, heals energy tears; soothes, calms, gives a profound sense of relief

ALLAMANDA
(Allamanda cathartica)

(Transpersonal Point) Purple

> **Add Gemstones:** Sugilite, Rutile Amethyst, Canadian Amethyst, Amethyst with Hematite, Selenite, Charoite, Violet Tourmaline, White Moonstone, Herkimer Diamond, Danburite
>
> Aids in recognizing and living spiritual truth, cleanses and heals the spiritual body, promotes opening and validating one's spirituality, provides all-aura cleansing and healing; helps in accessing highest level Light Be-ing guidance from angels, spirit guides, Goddess, Lords of Karma, etc.; amplifies psychic abilities and impressions, provides spiritual certainty and inner peace

ALLAMANDA
(Allamanda cathartica)

(Solar Plexus) Yellow

> **Add Gemstones:** Citrine, Amber Calcite, Golden Topaz, Golden Apophyllite, Amber, Yellow Fluorite, Yellow Zincite, Yellow Jade, Clear Quartz Crystal, Danburite
>
> Primary essence for cleansing, clearing and detoxifying, can be used in a sprayer to clear crystals and altars; emotional support for changing negative habits, supports ending addictions of all kinds (to drugs, alcohol, smoking, food addictions, addiction to a person); supports those working to end obsessions and obsessive behaviors; provides emotional clarity, reveals inner truth

ALLIUM
(Allium caeruleum)
(Throat) Blue

> **Add Gemstones:** Azurite, Lapis Lazuli, Blue Sapphire, Blue Aventurine, Azurite-Chrysocolla, Sodalite, Shattuckite, Iolite, Phenacite, Herkimer Diamond, Danburite
>
> Clears, heals and opens the throat chakra and throat complex (throat on all levels); promotes expression of one's inner truth on all levels, aids speaking out and speaking one's needs; good essence for channelers, teachers, singers, promotes all creativity; stimulates telepathy and animal communication abilities and promotes communication with spirit guides, angels, Lords of Karma, Goddess; opens, heals and clears the template doorways between the energy bodies; promotes positive transformation and change that may be intensive. Allium is also called Flowering Onion.

AMARYLLIS, Aphrodite
(Hippeastrum sp.)
(Heart) Pink and White

> **Add Gemstones:** Pink Garnet, Pink Andean Opal, Gem Rose Quartz, Pink Smithsonite, Lepidolite with Mica, Pink Calcite, Cobaltite, Herkimer Diamond, Danburite
>
> For finding love within oneself and without, draws in love of all kinds; supports relationships with soul mates and true friends, supports love between family members, supports love between parents and children; encourages positive self-love and the understanding of Goddess Within (that you are a Goddess in yourself); attracts divine love—love of the Goddesses and other Light Be-ings, promotes unconditional love both given and received; stimulates the awareness that you are loved.

AMARYLLIS, Best Seller
(Hippeastrum sp.)
(Heart) Pink

Add Gemstones: Pink Kunzite, Rhodochrosite, Rose Quartz, Dolomite, Pink Calcite, Pink Sapphire, Pink Chinese Opal, Pink Coral, Herkimer Diamond, Danburite

Provides emotional support for babies, children and their mothers; eases pregnant women's fears of birth and motherhood, supports women in labor for strength and easy childbirth; helps children adjust to Earth without losing the knowledge of who they really are, heals children's distress and disappointment; calms, soothes, stabilizes, reassures

AMARYLLIS, Blossom Peacock
(Hippeastrum sp.)
(Heart) Pink

Add Gemstones: Pink Tourmaline, Watermelon Tourmaline, Pink Sapphire, Cobaltite, Morganite, Lepidolite, Purple Kunzite, Selenite, Herkimer Diamond, Danburite

Clears and heals the heart chakra, the heart complex (heart chakras and channels through all the levels), and the emotional body through all levels; repairs and rewires the silver cord that connects one to life, heals damage to the silver cord; regenerates and heals karmic emotional damage begun in this lifetime; mends relationships and broken hearts, brings true soul mates together; heals grief

AMARYLLIS, Christmas Gift
(Hippeastrum sp.)
(Crown) White

>**Add Gemstones:** Yellow Topaz, Champagne Topaz, Citrine, Lemon Yellow Calcite, Dravite (Golden Tourmaline), Golden Labradorite, Yellow Opal, Herkimer Diamond, Danburite

>Fills the energy bodies with Light, fills the kundalini line and kundalini chakras with Light and cleansing; cleanses and purifies the aura and energy bodies; protects, repairs and heals; increases connection with Goddess in all Her forms, increases connection with the Light and all Light Be-ings; promotes faith and trust in life and in the Goddess/Light; increases clarity of thought and emotion, stimulates all mental processes and the mental body, provides all-healing

AMARYLLIS, Red Sensation
(Hippeastrum sp.)
(Root) Red

>**Add Gemstones:** Garnet, Moroccan Red Quartz, Canadian Amethyst with Hematite, Ruby, Star Ruby, Red Obsidian, Apache Tears Obsidian, Tektite, Clear Quartz Crystal, Danburite

>Supports and assists sexual love and union, fosters sexual compatibility, encourages joyful and responsible sexuality; aids true mates and lovers, encourages fulfilled marriages and domestic unions; aids the sexual expression of real love, supports life mates and the daily life of long term relationships; offers emotional support for sexual fears, sexual dysfunction, orgasm, and difficulties in conceiving a wanted child

AMARYLLIS, Rilona
(Hippeastrum sp.)
(Belly) Peach

>**Add Gemstones:** Peach Moonstone, Mexican Opal, Jelly Opal, Peach Sunstone, Honey Calcite, Peach Aventurine, Poppy Carnelian, Mookite, Clear Quartz Crystal, Danburite
>
>Helps a woman adjust on all levels to the idea of giving birth and motherhood, provides support for choosing to have a child; emotional support for fertility, conception, pregnancy and childbirth; heals the karmic connections between mother, father and child; heals the karmic and emotional blocks to fertility, conception and successful delivery; an emotional stabilizer for mothers-to-be, also supports women who try and fail to conceive

AMARYLLIS, Toronto
(Hippeastrum sp.)
(Belly) Orange and White

>**Add Gemstones:** Jacinth (Orange Sapphire), Peach Calcite, Mexican Opal, Jelly Opal, Amber, Brown Jasper, Red Phantom Calcite, Pecos Quartz, Clear Quartz Crystal, Danburite
>
>Stimulates the life force, increases the desire and will to be alive; general energy stimulant, sexual stimulant, increases and stimulates all healing on all levels; repairs and activates the hara chakra; increases the will to achieve one's life purpose, aids in defining one's life purpose, facilitates manifesting one's life purpose; heals lethargy, apathy, procrastination, speeds and warms

AMARYLLIS, Green Goddess
(Hippeastrum sp.)

(Diaphragm) Green

> **Add Gemstones:** Chrysoprase, Green Tourmaline, Peridot, Green Jade, Moldavite, Dioptase, Diopside, Green Aventurine, Green Amber, Green Zincite, Herkimer Diamond, Danburite
>
> Clears, repairs, heals, and cleanses the hara line chakras and channels and the emotional body; releases and removes karmic obstructions to the hara line; reprograms the emotions for joy and wellness, balances and stabilizes the emotions; can bring about a strong emotional release in the clearing; calms anger and resentment, promotes acceptance and a positive outlook, clears negativity of all sorts

AMARYLLIS, Grand Trumpet
(Hippeastrum sp.)

(Crown) White

> **Add Gemstones:** Larimar, Turquoise, Aquamarine, Amazonite, Blue Andean Opal, Blue Opal, Blue Chalcedony, Celestite, Herkimer Diamond, Danburite
>
> Repairs and opens the crown chakra, rewires and reprograms, cleanses and heals, removes obstructions and blockages, clears karmic patterns; heals and releases old karma with regard to thwarted or misused spirituality, offers another chance at becoming an enlightened Be-ing; heals and releases karma regarding serious misdeeds in past lifetimes, offers a new start and a clean slate; helps to prevent repeating old errors and thereby restoring the karma, inspires serious responsibility and learning a new way

ANEMONE
(Anemone coronaria de caen)

(Belly) Orange

Add Gemstones: Carnelian Agate, Carnelian, Poppy Carnelian, Peach Moonstone, Red Aventurine, Red Coral, Vanadinite, Clear Quartz Crystal, Danburite

Helps women who resent being female, who resent the menstrual cycle, and who resent women's roles; emotional support for all the issues of being female in a still sexist world, strengthens women to break the glass ceiling, promotes women's success in business and in life; balances the menstrual cycles by discouraging women from fighting normal menstrual processes; aids young women in menarche, supports older women entering menopause; emotional support for ovulation and conception, endometriosis, fibroids, menstrual pain, PMS

ANEMONE
(Anemone coronaria de caen)

(Heart) Pink

Add Gemstones: Pink Smithsonite, Pink Calcite, Pink Sapphire, Gem Rose Quartz, Pink Druzy Quartz, Pink Spirit Quartz, Clear Quartz Crystal, Danburite

Promotes trust in life and in the universe, allows one to "let go and let Goddess" and trust in the Light; heals raw emotions, soothes and calms the emotions, cleanses the heart chakra; helps heartache, heartbreak, grief, heart-loss; promote acceptance, encourages moving forward, helps in returning joy to one's life, aids in finding and keeping new hope; encourages new things to hold one's interest and to give life meaning

ANEMONE
(Anemone coronaria de caen)

(Crown) Purple

> **Add Gemstones:** Amethyst, Rutile Amethyst, Violet Tourmaline, Alexandrite, Selenite, Phenacite, Girasol Quartz, Clear Quartz Crystal, Danburite
>
> Supports soothing sleep, aids insomnia and restlessness by reducing stress, reduces mental chatter; offers the Light's protection from nightmares and night terrors, offers the Light's guidance out of and into body; promotes lucid dreaming, helps in remembering and learning from dreams, provides healing dreams, aids spiritual dreamwork; supports and protects those who do astral travel awake or asleep by providing increased protection

ANEMONE
(Anemone coronaria de caen)

(All-Aura) White

> **Add Gemstones:** White Moonstone, White Apophyllite, Selenite, White Jade, White Stillbite, Rainbow Moonstone, Herkimer Diamond, Clear Quartz Crystal, Danburite
>
> Soothes and stabilizes the aura and etheric (closest to physical) energy body, balances the kundalini chakras; cleanses, clears and repairs the aura, chakras and etheric body; heals holes, tears and rips in the auric envelope; fills the aura with Light and love, promotes trust in the Light and the Goddess; energy protector and purifier; promotes clarity and optimism, encourages inner peace, emotionally soothing and calming

ANGEL TRUMPET
(Brugmansia suaveolens)

(Transpersonal Point) Peach

Add Gemstones: Chrysoberyl, Chrysoberyl Catseye, Diaspor, Labradorite, Rainbow Moonstone, Phenacite, Selenite, Champagne Topaz, Herkimer Diamond, Danburite

Aid to accessing star wisdom and wisdom from other planets and dimensions; promotes connection with Pleiadians, other-planetary healers and helpers, increases connection to Goddess (especially Star Goddesses), star guides, spirit guides; encourages channeling, increases spiritual awareness of all kinds; initiates and increases soul level healing and core soul healing, repairs the DNA

ANGEL TRUMPET
(Brugmansia sp.)

(Heart) Pink

Add Gemstones: Pink Sapphire, Pink Tourmaline, Pink Kunzite, Pink Calcite, Clear Calcite, Selenite, Phenacite, Herkimer Diamond, Danburite

Clears and heals all emotional heart pain, repairs and reconnects, regenerates damage from this life and past lives; heals the heart on all levels (heart complex), and all heart-related energetic systems (the chakras of the thymus, breasts, hands, and the emotional and higher emotional levels); heals the Higher Self and brings her into conscious connection; increases one's conscious connection with angelic realm protectors; encourages a healed heart, encourages a joyful heart and a joyful life

ANGEL TRUMPET
(Brugmansia sp.)
(Transpersonal Point) White

> **Add Gemstones:** Angel Wing Selenite, Clear Tourmaline, White Moonstone, Grey Moonstone, Angelite, Phenacite, Seraphanite, Azurite, Clear Quartz Crystal, Danburite
>
> Enhances one's connection with spirit guides, Goddess, angels, Lords of Karma, helper aliens and other positive discarnate teachers and Light Be-ings; accesses star wisdom and other-planetary wisdom, increases psychic communication and reception of all types; promotes and increases the psychic ability to channel, supports and strengthens mediumship, enhances meditation, protects astral travel, strengthens psychic healing; increases spiritual awareness and evolution, aids soul level healing, repairs damaged DNA

ANGEL TRUMPET, Nightblooming
(Brugmansia inoxia)
(Transpersonal Point) White

> **Add Gemstones:** All white stones—White Moonstone, Rutilated Quartz Crystal, Snow Quartz, White Calcite, White Phantom Quartz, Phenacite, Clear Quartz Crystal, Herkimer Diamond, Danburite
>
> Promotes dreaming, lucid dreams, dream remembrance, and all aspects of spiritual dreamwork; stimulates prophetic and healing dreams, helps in understanding and using dreams and dream symbolism, aids in contacting psychic guides in the dream state; reduces insomnia, deepens sleep states; promotes psychic opening and spiritual evolution, increases psychic awareness and ability to dream

ANGEL TRUMPET DATURA
(Datura metel)

(Crown) Purple

> **Add Gemstones:** Charoite, Sugilite, Alexandrite, Amethyst, Rutile Amethyst, Purple Fluorite, Lepidolite, Tanzanite, Herkimer Diamond, Danburite
>
> Provides understanding of the wheel of birth, death and rebirth; enhances understanding of reincarnation and past lifetimes; aids in past life regression, soul journeys, helps in learning to work with the Lords of Karma for karmic release and healing; provides maximum karmic evolution, soul growth and positive transformation; promotes karmic grace and core soul healing, repairs the DNA; good support for old souls, incarnated bodhisattvas and soul mate unions; helps those in service to the Light to avoid despair and burnout

ANGEL TRUMPET DATURA
(Datura metel)

(Solar Plexus) Yellow

> **Add Gemstones:** Yellow Opal, Golden Beryl, Topaz, Selenite, Yellow Fluorite, Yellow Sunstone, Clear Lemon Calcite, Golden Labradorite, Clear Quartz Crystal, Danburite
>
> Promotes opening one's consciousness to angels, plant and animal devas, gemstone spirits, planetary guardians, and other-planetary helpers and healers; facilitates the ability to perceive and communicate with nonphysical life forms and spirits; aids those who wish to learn from fairies and other nonphysical Be-ings; helps in the psychic sending and receiving of visual images and ideas, aids in channeling and automatic writing of received information; provides connection with Goddesses and Light Be-ings, brings in Light energy, promotes core soul healing, cleanses and purifies, increases clarity

ANISE HYSSOP
(Agastache foeniculum)

(Throat) Blue

Add Gemstones: Shattukite, Blue Siberian Quartz, Blue Kyanite, Natural Star Sapphire, Lapis Lazuli, Celestite, Larimar, Blue Chalcedony, Herkimer Diamond, Danburite

An essence for understanding and living in truth, promotes one's ability to recognize truth, encourages being always truthful; increases one's ability to know one's personal inner truths and to live by them, encourages the speaking out of one's personal truths and all truth; encourages integrity and honesty in everything one does and thinks; good for those who have avoided hard truths, good for those who now recognize hard truths and choose to heal their lives; helps to make one an advocate for those who have no power or voice in society and in their own lives; an essence for truth and integrity on every level

ANISE HYSSOP, Heather Queen
(Agastache heather queen)

(Causal Body) Deep Pink

Add Gemstones: Lepidolite, Lepidolite with Rubellite, Rose Aura Crystal, Pink Fluorite, Stichtite, Pink Sapphire, Purple Kunzite, Raspberry Garnet, Pink Tourmaline, Herkimer Diamond, Danburite

Promotes an understanding of spiritual truth, promotes receiving spiritual teaching and information; gives one the ability to receive spirituality teachings and pass them on to others, offers clarity and understanding of information received, offers putting spiritual information into earth plane perspective; brings in teachers of the Light—angels, spirit guides, other-planet helpers, Lords of Karma, devas—willing to instruct and teach; promotes connection with Goddess and the Light; heals the inability to recognize truth and receive it

AZALEA
(Rhododendron sp.)

(Heart) Pink

> **Add Gemstones:** Cobaltite, Pink Sapphire, Lepidolite, Lepidolite with Rubellite, Pink Andean Opal, Rose Quartz, Phenacite, Clear Quartz Crystal, Danburite

> Heals past life and this life emotional wounds to the heart chakra, heals the heart complex (heart on all levels) and aura layers, provides karmic healing for the emotional body; opens the heart to receiving and giving love and forgiveness, heals heart scars by dissolving them gently, repairs and reconnects nonphysical heart anatomy; increases the soul's participation in the physical body, supports physical heart healing

AZALEA
(Rhododendron sp.)

(Crown) White

> **Add Gemstones:** Purple Fluorite, Aquamarine, Elestial Quartz, Phenacite, Violet Tourmaline, Charoite, Seraphanite, Clear Quartz Crystal, Herkimer Diamond, Danburite

> Promotes ascension (enlightenment) the union of body and soul, the joining of the physical body with the soul bodies, Goddess realization or Goddess within; promotes inner knowing and inner peace, increases and supports spirituality and spiritual evolution, aids inner growth and healing; increases connection with the Goddess and with one's soul, increases connection with spiritual guides and guidance; aids mediumship and channeling, meditation, aids all spiritual work

BABY HAWAIIAN ROSEWOOD
(Argyreia nervosa)
(Third Eye) Blue-Lavender

Add Gemstones: Holly Blue Agate, Larimar, Blue Tourmaline, Lapis Lazuli, Sugilite, Azurite, Blue Aventurine, Amethyst, Blue Fluorite, Herkimer Diamond, Danburite

For spiritual growth and transformation; stimulates prophecy and clairvoyance, stimulates channeling, increases and opens all psychic skills and abilities, promotes new psychic opening; aids and protects psychics from energy attacks and attachments, heals the damage from psychic attacks and negative interference; clears energy channels and chakras, prevents the taking on of others' symptoms or negativity, dissolves negativity; clears and purifies

BEE BALM
(Monarda didymaby)
(Root) Red

Add Gemstones: Hematite, Red Obsidian, Rainbow Obsidian, Black Onyx, Chrysanthymum Stone, Zebra Jasper, Black Tourmaline, Clear Quartz Crystal, Danburite

For grounding into the physical, brings one's energy fully into the earth plane and into incarnation; heals the grounding cord and grounding system, connects the grounding cord properly to the core of the Earth; prevents unwanted astral travel or out of body travel; reduces uncontrolled psychic impressions and spaciness, slows psychic opening for those afraid of it and eases the fear; reduces flightiness, daydreaming, irresponsiblity, lack of concentration and improper silliness. Also called Scarlet Balm or Oswego Tea

BIRD OF PARADISE
(Strelitzia reginae)(Hara)

Orange and Blue

> **Add Gemstones:** Amber, Jelly Opal, Mexican Opal, Blue Opal, Blue Andean Opal, Fire Opal, White Opal, Black Opal, Clear Quartz Crystal, Danburite

> For focusing the knowledge and intent of one's life purpose, brings the spirituality of one's life purpose into physical manifestation and everyday living; expands the hara line and kundalini line channels and chakras, cleanses and clears the hara line, releases obstructions to the hara line and to realizing one's life purpose; helps women in abused relationships to break free; protects free will and personal freedom, promotes rapid energy expansion and spiritual evolution

BIRD OF PARADISE
(Strelitzia reginae)

(Heart) White

> **Add Gemstones:** Pink Sapphire, Kunzite, Pink Tourmaline, White Phantom Quartz, Selenite, Phenacite, Natrolite, Mother of Pearl, Clear Quartz Crystal, Danburite

> Inspires the heart taking wings; clears and repairs the silver cord that keeps one connected to life; heals and aligns the energy bodies and the connections between energy bodies; promotes the anchoring in of the Higher Self, Essence Self and Goddess Self in ascension processes (Essential Energy Balancing); facilitates ascension and all ascension processes for enlightenment (ascension) in this lifetime; offers emotional and spiritual transformation; promotes energy purification and clarity

BLANKET FLOWER
(Galliardia grandiflora)

(Belly) Orange

> **Add Gemstones:** Honey Calcite, Champagne Topaz, Orange Calcite, Jacinth (Orange Sapphire), Zincite, Amber, Mexican Opal, Jelly Opal, Herkimer Diamond, Danburite
>
> Warms and comforts, cheers, inspires security and the feeling that everything is alright, inspires confidence in oneself and others; promotes the feeling of being able to handle whatever situation has arisen or will arise; helps one to find and use the competence that is waiting within; helps with being calm in a storm and knowing just what to do, makes one into the person others can depend upon; a good essence for mothers who must always know how

BLEEDING HEART
(Clerodendrum thomsoniae)

(Causal Body) Red and White

> **Add Gemstones:** Garnet, White Moonstone, Ruby, Star Ruby, Spinel, Clear Kunzite, Clear Beryl, Clear Tourmaline, Diamond, Clear Quartz Crystal, Danburite
>
> Supports and heals the bodhisattvas—the healers and planetary servers—those who give too much of themselves for others' sake; heals burnout, depletion, exhaustion, depression and despair; offers hope, strength and grounding in the now, aids regeneration and energy healing, restores strength and the ability to keep on giving

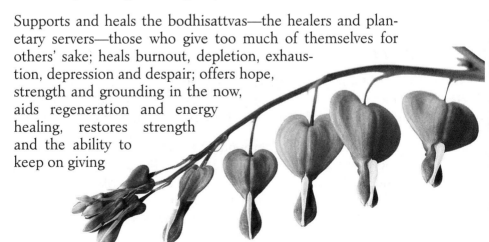

BLUEBIRD VINE
— *See PETRA VINE*

GINGER, Blue
(Dichorisandra thyrsiflora)
(Throat) Blue

> **Add Gemstones:** Larimar, Lapis Lazuli, Blue Lace Agate, Amazonite, Blue Aventurine, Angelite, Blue Calcite, Sodalite, Clear Quartz Crystal, Danburite
>
> Aids the ability to speak out, helps in recognizing and expressing one's needs, helps in meeting one's needs and taking care of oneself; promotes positive assertiveness; a good essence for those who speak out against societal wrongs and those who protect the innocent—social workers, public defenders, child abuse workers, etc.; helps those recovering from violent victimization (rape, mugging, physical attack, incest, battering); promotes creativity and self-healing of all types, clears the throat. Blue ginger is not actually a member of the ginger family.

BOTTLE BRUSH TREE
(Callisteman lanceolatus)
(Root) Red

> **Add Gemstones:** Red Spinel, Garnet, Red Moroccan Quartz, Pecos Quartz, Red Phantom Quartz, Red Jasper, Red Obsidian, Red Coral, Clear Quartz Crystal, Danburite
>
> For connecting one's grounding cord properly with the core of the Earth, brings one fully into the body; provides grounding and centering, establishes stability and security, offers sense of physical safety, promotes responsibility in one's actions, facilitates physical independence; enables letting go because you are now securely connected

BOUGAINVILLEA
(Bougainvillea sp.)

(Heart) Fuchsia

Add Gemstones: Pink Tourmaline, Red Moroccan Quartz, Garnet, Raspberry Garnet, Pink Sapphire, Pink Calcite, Red Spinel, Ruby, Herkimer Diamond, Danburite

Creates, repairs and enhances the connections and interconnections of body, emotions, mind and spirit; heals the bodies separately and together; aids emotional body healing, opens and heals the heart chakra; promotes being an individual and expressing one's individuality, enhances free expression and creativity; promotes balance and inner harmony, fosters sensitivity and inner peace

BOUGAINVILLEA
(Bougainvillea sp.)

(Heart) Light Pink

Add Gemstones: Rose Quartz, Gem Rose Quartz, Pink Kunzite, Lepidolite, Cobaltite, Pink Andean Opal, Pink Coral, Selenite, Clear Quartz Crystal, Danburite

Aids birth and giving birth, provides a welcome to the world, soothes infants and new mothers, helps to bring the newborn's soul into the body; aids physical, emotional and spiritual growth for mother and baby; aids bonding of mother and baby

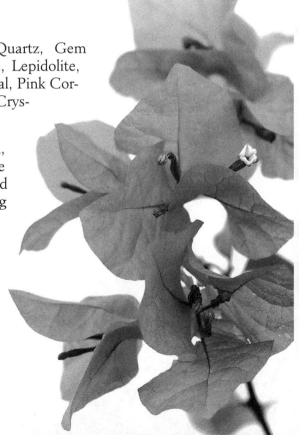

BOUGAINVILLEA
(Bougainvillea sp.)

(Transpersonal Point) White

> **Add Gemstones:** Fresh Water Pearl, White Opal, White Moonstone, Rainbow Moonstone, Clear Kunzite, Clear Beryl, Clear Fluorite, Herkimer Diamond, Danburite
>
> Eases the process and promotes the acceptance of aging, change and death; supports a joyful old age, aids in trusting the processes of life and age, promotes wisdom and growth; supports emotional transformations, eases and aids the death transition; helps in connecting with spirit guides, angels and the Goddess; reduces stress, promotes inner peace

BROMELIAD
(Aechmea fasciata)

(Heart) Pink

> **Add Gemstones:** Pink Kunzite, Rhodochrosite, Raspberry Garnet, Rose Quartz, Pink Tourmaline, Watermelon Tourmaline, Pink Smithsonite, Herkimer Diamond, Danburite
>
> For unfolding and releasing old secrets of the heart, aids healing and moving forward, facilitates healing past pain that remains and festers, promotes emotional release and emotional resolution; also heals grief, shame, resentment, anger, blame and self-blame; assists in letting go, promotes forgiveness of others and oneself; encourages speaking out about hurt that has long been held within, promotes finishing and completing old emotional pain. Also called Silver Urn Plant

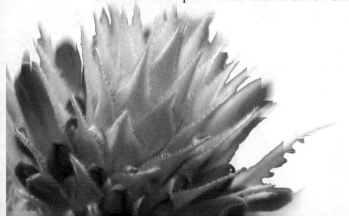

BROMELIAD
(Tillsandia)

(Root) Red

> **Add Gemstones:** Ruby, Spinel, Red Obsidian, Rainbow Obsidian, Hematite, Black Tourmaline, Garnet, Moroccan Red Quartz, Clear Quartz Crystal, Danburite
>
> Transforms and heals anger, releases rage safely, eases resentment, reduces depression; strengthens the life force and will to live, promotes compassion for oneself and others; provides emotional support for those with debilitating, life threatening or chronic dis-eases, raises hope

BUDDLEIA
— *See BUTTERFLY BUSH*

BUTTERCUP
(Ranunculus acris)

(Solar Plexus) Yellow

> **Add Gemstones:** Golden Topaz, Golden Calcite, Yellow Jade, Yellow Fluorite, Golden Beryl, Natural Citrine, Golden Amber, Clear Quartz Crystal, Danburite
>
> Promotes cleansing, clearing and releasing; catalyzes inner change, promotes inner growth, eases life's transitions; activates and escalates energy flows (ch'i) through the nonphysical and physical bodies; supports energy changes and shifts, aligns the energy bodies; develops, clears and opens the higher level energy bodies; promotes assimilation in all forms (physical food and nourishment, mental ideas, energy), calms

BUTTERFLY BUSH
Adonis Blue (Buddleia davidii)

(Third Eye) Blue

> **Add Gemstones:** Shattuckite, Blue Sapphire, Blue Quartz, Blue Opal, Lapis Lazuli, Blue Chalcedony, Dumortierite, Blue Aventurine, Sodalite, Herkimer Diamond, Danburite
>
> Clears the third eye of karmic obstructions and obstructions from core soul damage, removes karmic blocks to the third eye, purifies and cleanses; opens the karma that has been too painful to see for the purpose of releasing and healing it; stimulates and causes past life visions, initiates spontaneous karmic release visions; promote working with the Lords of Karma, accelerates the release of old karma, accelerates spiritual growth; can open a flood of visions and accelerated psychic experiences, provides necessary healing but may not do so gently

BUTTERFLY BUSH, Bicolor
(Buddleia x weyeriana)

(Heart and Solar Plexus) Yellow and Pink

> **Add Gemstones:** Rhodochrosite, Gem Rhodochrosite, Yellow Topaz, Ametrine, Natural Citrine, Pink Calcite, Pink Tourmaline, Amber, Clear Quartz Crystal, Danburite
>
> Connects and balances the heart with the solar plexus, connects physicality with spirituality; changes love into unconditional love, energy into Light, thought into service to the Light; brings heart energy into the mind and mental logic into the emotions, helps those who are too soft emotionally or too much "in their heads"; balances cold mental logic with caring and compassion—good essence for scientists, doctors and nurses; balances over emotionality with clear thought; inspires compassion

BUTTERFLY BUSH, Black Knight
(Buddleia davidi)

(Earth) Purple-Black

Add Gemstones: Sugilite, Charoite, Violet Tourmaline, Black Tourmaline, Black Velvet Tourmaline, Purple Obsidian, Black Jade, Clear Quartz Crystal, Danburite

Promotes acceptance of what cannot be changed and must be; fosters determination for positive change in one's life, supports through processes of change and healing; provides stability in times of transition and transformation, stabilizes in times of uprooting; transforms negative habits and addictions; connects one to the planet, makes one's hold on life secure, promotes feeling secure; centers, grounds and stabilizes; heals grief, encourages calm and inner peace

BUTTERFLY BUSH, Honeycomb
(Buddleia x weyeriana)

(Solar Plexus) Yellow

Add Gemstones: Yellow Sunstone, Yellow Jade, Yellow Topaz, Natural Citrine, Yellow Sapphire, Golden Beryl, Golden Labradorite, Lemon Yellow Calcite, Herkimer Diamond, Danburite

Fills the kundalini chakras and channels with Light and healing, fills the aura and auric field with Light, repairs tears and rips in chakras and aura; promotes core soul healing at the mental body level, releases negative entities and removes obstructions; brings optimism, mental quiet, mental peace, relief; offers calm and healing after stress and trauma, heals after times of great endurance and upset, shows the Light at the end of the tunnel

BUTTERFLY WEED
(Asclepias tuberosa)

(Hara) Orange

> **Add Gemstones:** Orange Sunstone, Jelly Opal, Carnelian, Carnelian Agate, Vanadinite, Amber, Mookite, Orange Calcite, Honey Calcite, Herkimer Diamond, Danburite
>
> For finding one's wings and ability to fly; promotes spiritual freedom, psychic flight, astral travel, meditation, shamanic journeys, star journeys; aids retrieval of soul fragments, core soul healing, repair of DNA; increases one's awareness of lifetimes on other planets or in other galaxies, promotes contacting one's inner wisdom and the wisdom of the Earth and other planets, stimulates awareness of and beyond Earth consciousness

BUTTERFLY WEED
(Asclepias tuberosa)

(Root) Red

> **Add Gemstones:** Vanadinite, Red Aventurine, Red Jade, Ruby, Star Ruby, Garnet, Spinel, Cuprite, Mexican Fire Opal, Herkimer Diamond, Danburite
>
> Brings one back to Earth after flights of fancy or astral travel, brings the sites from other places into one's life at home; stimulates the life force and increases the flow of Earth energy through the chakras and kundalini line; promotes core soul healing of the energy channels and flows, heals the connections between chakras, repairs the DNA; inspires joy and passion, intensity, living life to the fullest; balances the urge to travel with remembering to come home

CALENDULA
—*See MARIGOLD*

CALIFORNIA POPPY
(Eschscholzia californica)

(Root) Red

> **Add Gemstones:** Garnet, Ruby, Moroccan Red Quartz, Amethyst with Hematite, Red Pietersite, Spinel, Red Siberian Quartz, Clear Quartz Crystal, Danburite
>
> Heals, increases and stabilizes the life force, increases the will to live and to continue with one's life, heals despair and not wanting to be here; brings the soul force into the physical body levels, offers an emotional jump-start for those in danger of giving up, good remedy for fragile new infants and the critically ill or depressed; increases vitality and hope

CALLA LILY, Cameo
(Zantedeschia rehmannii superba)

(Third Eye) Cream

> **Add Gemstones:** Peach Moonstone, White Moonstone, Grey Moonstone, Peach Aventurine, White Jade, Dolomite, Mother of Pearl, Poppy Carnelian, Clear Quartz Crystal, Danburite
>
> Promotes making magick and ritual, aids in changing consciousness at will, increases one's connection to Goddess; supports priestesses and ritual planners, good High Priestess essence; good essence for anyone focusing on feminine spirituality or the Moon Goddesses; psychic opener, helps maintain meditation states, helps those who do dreamwork to remember and record their dreams, increases understanding of psychic images and happenings, aids any psychic work

CALLA LILY, Captain Eskimo
(Zantedeschia aethiopica)

(Hara) Yellow

Add Gemstones: Champagne Topaz, Amber, Honey Calcite, Yellow Jade, Rutile Citrine, Sunstone, Yellow Kyanite, Yellow Apatite, Herkimer Diamond, Danburite

Cleanses, clears and purifies the hara line energy channels; removes blockages and obstructions to personal and spiritual growth; provides all-aura cleansing and purification, fills the aura with Light and healing; supports the path to enlightenment (ascension) and all positive spiritual evolutionary paths, aids in manifesting one's life purpose easily and successfully

CALLA LILY, Captain Palermo
(Zantedeschia sp.)

(Earth) Black

Add Gemstones: Black Tourmaline, Smoky Quartz, Black Star Sapphire, Hematite, Amethyst with Hematite, Black Pearl, Clear Quartz Crystal, Danburite

Promotes connection to the Earth, supports being in body as a part of this planet; provides rootedness in the planet, connects one's grounding cord properly into the Earth's core, repairs the grounding cord and system; encourages stability and seriousness, increases a sense of responsibility and mission toward the Earth; good essence for planetary healers and those who help and heal life on Earth, good essence for those who work with animals (domestic, pets, wildlife); helps those who are not grounded enough, helps those who do not know their place or life purpose for this incarnation

CALLA LILY, Dwarf Pink
(Zantedeschia rehmannii superba)

(Heart) Pink

> **Add Gemstones:** Pink Coral, Rose Quartz, Morganite, Pink Kunzite, Lepidolite with Rubellite, Pink Smithsonite, Pink Calcite, Pink Jade, Herkimer Diamond, Danburite
>
> Supports and promotes fertility, conception, pregnancy, labor, delivery, breast feeding, and childbirth recovery for mother and infant; emotional support and strengthener for the problems of pregnancy, miscarriage, postpartum depression, exhaustion and debility; good infant essence, helps newborns adjust to life on Earth; aid to midwives, also offers emotional comfort and recovery after abortion

CALLA LILY, Flame
(Zantedeschia rehmanni superba)

(Root) Orange

> **Add Gemstones:** Red Jasper, Red Coral, Red Aventurine, Mexican Opal, Jelly Opal, Moroccan Red Quartz, Peach Moonstone, White Moonstone, Clear Quartz Crystal, Danburite
>
> Aids women in taking their power, promotes women's emotional strength, positive assertiveness, ability to say no to bad relationships and situations, recognizing and avoiding unsafe men; aids recovery from abuse, incest, rape and battering; promotes self-love, positive self-worth, healthy self-image, positive body image and take-charge strength

CALLA LILY, Giant White
(Zantedeschia aethiopica)

(Third Eye) White

> **Add Gemstones:** Azurite, Azurite-Chrysocolla, Blue Tourmaline, Blue Aventurine, Sodalite, Lapis Lazuli, Blue Sapphire, Blue Dumortierite, Iolite, Herkimer Diamond, Danburite
>
> Cleanses, clears and purifies the mental body and mental body chakras; removes mental blocks to personal and spiritual growth, removes negative thought forms and beliefs, aids in healing negative karmic patterns; stimulates psychic development and increases psychic strength, increases psychic information received and the ability to understand it; promotes psychic healing ability, clairvoyance, telepathy, channeling, crystal ball gazing, meditation and other psychic skills

CALLA LILY, Lavender Gem
(Zantedeschia sp.)

(Crown) Lavender

> **Add Gemstones:** Rutile Amethyst, Amethyst, Canadian Amethyst, Violet Tourmaline, Sugilite, Purple Dumortierite, Violet Jade, Phenacite, Herkimer Diamond, Danburite
>
> Promotes faith in life's processes, increases one's trust in the divine, brings spirituality into one's life and awareness, offers the understanding that there is a purpose in all things and in all lives; heals crises of faith for those of all religions, transcends all religions, aids depression, heals despair

CALLA LILY, Naomi Campbell
(Zantedeschia sp.)
(Grounding) Purple-Black

Add Gemstones: Rainbow Obsidian, Purple Obsidian, Purple Dumortierite, Black Tourmaline, Amethyst with Hematite, Tourmaline Quartz, Onyx, Clear Quartz Crystal, Danburite

Connects the Earth and the Sky, the Above and Below; brings the spiritual into the physical and grounds the physical fully into the planet; good essence for those who teach spirituality and need grounded information and explanations, brings nonphysical teaching into physical comprehension; opens the crown and the grounding system, opens the entire kundalini line, heals and repairs, balances and stabilizes; makes one's physical life spiritual, makes one's spiritual life physical; promotes full connectedness to the planet without sacrificing psychic opening; enhances all psychic abilities, promotes spiritual evolution

CALLA LILY, Treasure
(Zantedeschia rehmanii superba)
(Belly) Orange

Add Gemstones: Tangerine Quartz, Mexican Opal, Jelly Opal, Peach Moonstone, Peach Calcite, Amber, Peach Aventurine, Sunstone, Feldspar, Clear Quartz Crystal, Danburite

Aids those who work with the fairy realm; increases the psychic ability to see, hear and speak with fairies, devas, plant and tree spirits, garden spirits, gemstone spirits; promotes recognizing and learning from the small invisible lives that ordain nature; helps with learning about co-creation and co-operation with nature and nature spirits; also helps in communicating with and working with animal spirits and totem animals

CAMELLIA, Donation
(Camellia x williamsii)

(Crown) Lavender

> **Add Gemstones:** Purple Kunzite, Lepidolite with Mica, Pink Kunzite, Pink Fluorite, Pink Tourmaline, Violet Tourmaline, Amethyst, Alexandrite, Herkimer Diamond, Danburite
>
> Clears and heals the symptoms and discomforts of spiritual growth and expansion, aids the ascension process, fosters enlightenment, balances kundalini rising experiences; stabilizes, promotes integration, aids in trusting the Goddess and the process; regenerates, facilitates positive cellular repatterning, aids DNA clearing and repatterning, fills the aura with Light on all levels, expands the chakras and energy bodies; provides calm and peacefulness during change and transformation, accelerates spiritual evolution

CAMELLIA
(Camellia japonica)

(Heart) Pink

> **Add Gemstones:** Pink Kunzite, Morganite, Rose Quartz, Pink Jade, Pink Calcite, Cobaltite, Clear Beryl, Pink Coral, Dolomite, Clear Quartz Crystal, Danburite
>
> Brings healing and compassion into one's life--for oneself and to offer to others, and uses compassion to heal the heart; promotes forgiveness of oneself and others, fills the heart with compassion for all life, reminds of the oneness of all life, encourages unconditional love for oneself and others; promotes healthy self-esteem and respect for others, offers inner peace, calm certainty; an essence that invokes the Goddess, especially Kwan Yin and Tara

CAMELLIA
(Camellia japonica)

(Heart) Pink and White

Add Gemstones: Pink Tourmaline, Peach Moonstone, White Moonstone, Pink Fluorite, Rose Quartz, Pink Kunzite, Selenite, Phenacite, Herkimer Diamond, Danburite

Primarily focuses on healing the core soul of all damage; brings in, heals and integrates soul fragments; repairs and ends the damage of soul fragmentation on all levels; promotes spiritual growth and transformation; provides karmic grace and intervention for karmic healing, releases the karma so the core soul can be fully healed; provides connection with Mother Mary, the All-Mother, Goddesses and Gods, the Lords of Karma, devas, spirit guides and angels, other-planetary soul healers; repairs the DNA, provides inner peace and all-healing

CAMELLIA
(Camellia japonica)

(Root) Red

Add Gemstones: Garnet, Red Coral, Ruby, Star Ruby, Moroccan Red Quartz, Spinel, Red Pietersite, Red Obsidian, Black Tourmaline, Jet, Herkimer Diamond, Danburite

Heals lost love and draws new love in; heals grief, heartache, heartbreak, aids recovery from broken relationships, promotes ability to open to new love, stabilizes new relationships and unions, aids success in marriage and long term relationships, promotes compatible sexuality and lovers' bonding

CAMELLIA, White by the Gate
(Camellia japonica)
(Crown) White

> **Add Gemstones:** Selenite, Phenacite, White Apophyllite, Aragonite, Citrine, Golden Labradorite, Rainbow Moonstone, Herkimer Diamond, Danburite
>
> Provides karmic healing and repatterning, accesses karmic grace; clears, heals and opens all the energy bodies and chakras on all levels; fills all the energy bodies and levels with Light and peace; heals and releases negative and outmoded belief systems, changes negative thoughts and thought patterns to positive ones, clears all thinking that holds back spiritual growth and healing; increases connection with the Lords of Karma for karmic healing and accelerated spiritual growth; initiates core soul healing, repairs and heals DNA

CAMELLIA, Winter's Snowman
(Camellia japonica)
(Transpersonal Point) White

> **Add Gemstones:** White Phantom Quartz, White Opal, Fire Opal, Clear Beryl, White Moonstone, Rainbow Moonstone, Stilbite, Clear Quartz Crystal, Danburite
>
> For finding the Goddess and the Light, accessing spirit guides and angels; promotes finding the Goddess within oneself (Goddess Within), promotes contact with one's soul; helps to heal the higher energy bodies, initiates core soul healing and repair, heals soul fragmentation, heals the DNA; supports a spiritual path and the path to ascension (enlightenment); increases spiritual and psychic development, guides advanced psychic development and soul growth

CAMELLIA
(Camellia japonica)
(Solar Plexus) Yellow

Add Gemstones: Yellow Opal, Amber, Natural Citrine, Rutile Citrine, Golden Labradorite, Golden Beryl, Yellow Fluorite, Yellow Sapphire, Clear Quartz Crystal, Danburite

Brings in Light through all of the energy levels and bodies, provides psychic protection; clears the mental body, hara and kundalini channels and chakras of negative attachments, entities, implants and interference; provides core soul repair and healing, provides mind grid repair and healing, heals and repairs the DNA; good essence for those doing karmic release work

CANDLE BUSH
(Cassia alata)
(Hara) Yellow

Add Gemstones: Yellow Opal, Amber, Golden Beryl, Golden Topaz, Champagne Topaz, Dravite (Golden Tourmaline), Golden Apophyllite, Herkimer Diamond, Danburite

Lights a golden Light in the deepest darkness, illuminates, offers hope where there had been none, reveals the Light at the end of dark tunnels; invokes Goddess and the Light, brings in the help of Light Be-ings; cleanses, clears and purifies; provides cleansing for the chakras, energy bodies and channels; removes negative energy and interference, clears negative entities and attachments; helps negative-seeming people to "lighten up"

CANNA
(Canna generalis striatus)
(Hara) Red and Gold

> **Add Gemstones:** Mexican Opal, Amber, Red Jasper, Red Coral, Rhodochrosite, Jacinth (Orange Sapphire), Carnelian, Vanadinite, Clear Quartz Crystal, Danburite
>
> Fosters joy and love of life, increases vitality and the life force; offers knowledge of one's life purpose and the means to achieve it; supports joyful sexuality that is both physical and spiritual, enhances one's ability to see the good and joyful in everyone and everything; ends apathy, reduces sadness and depression, heals grief, promotes playfulness

CARDINAL CLIMBER VINE
(Ipomea sp.)
(Perineum) Red

> **Add Gemstones:** Moroccan Red Quartz, Mexican Opal, Garnet, Spinel, Red Jasper, Ruby, Amethyst with Hematite, Hematite, Clear Quartz Crystal, Danburite
>
> Manifests one's true life path onto the Earth and into physical reality, promotes finding one's life purpose and accomplishing it, strengthens the will to achieve one's life purpose; brings life force energy into the hara line channels, increases personal energy levels, promotes the circulation of ch'i (life energy); aids grounding and centering into daily reality, increases determination and the will to live, cleanses and purifies, calms and stabilizes

CASSIA TREE
(Cassia sp.)

(Solar Plexus) Yellow and Pink

> **Add Gemstones:** Natural Citrine, Pink Kunzite, Yellow Fluorite, Yellow Opal, Rhodochrosite, Yellow Calcite, Pink Calcite, Pink Jade, Rose Quartz, Clear Quartz Crystal, Danburite
>
> For balancing power in relationships; helps in resisting manipulation from others, aids in the divorce process, assists in leaving abusive or battering relationships, promotes reentry into single life and making one's living alone; helps to create the qualities of inner empowerment, self-confidence, healthy self-love, inner strength; helps one to see the Goddess within

CATTAIL
(Typha latifolia)

(Movement) Tan

> **Add Gemstones:** Petrified Wood, Ammonite Fossil, Ocean Jasper, Brecciated Jasper, Golden Leaf Jasper, Rainforest Jasper, Tiger Eye, Moldavite, Smoky Quartz, Clear Quartz Crystal, Danburite
>
> For moving forward in one's life and on one's spiritual path in a smooth and sustained manner; facilitates steady growth and forward progress, opens and releases blocks, overcomes obstacles and obstructions; connects the Earth and the Sky, connects the Above and Below, brings the physical and spiritual together and integrates them into a comfortable whole; makes one's earth plane life a spiritual life, grounds one's spiritual practice into everyday living and everyday earth plane reality; erases the separation between body and spirit, grounds and stabilizes, promotes success and prosperity

CENTAURY PLANT
(Agave amaericana)

(Hara) Orange

> **Add Gemstones:** Pecos Quartz, Red Phantom Quartz, Orange Zincite, Carnelian, Orange Agate, Honey Calcite, Orange Calcite, Amber, Clear Quartz Crystal, Danburite
>
> Provides the courage to follow one's life path despite any difficulty or criticism, increases awareness of life purpose, enhances strength of resolve, offers realistic self-awareness and estimate of what one can and cannot do; helps to end victimization and abusive situations, helps to heal from abuse in this life and past lives, aids one's ability to leave an abuser, releases anger

CHALICE VINE
(Solandra nitida zucs) (Perineum)

Maroon and Cream

> **Add Gemstones:** Canadian Amethyst, Garnet, Black Opal, Ruby, Star Ruby, Amethyst with Hematite, Hematite, Black Tourmaline, Red Obsidian, Clear Quartz Crystal, Danburite
>
> Represents and heals the sacred feminine, the sacred womb; promotes transmission of the life force from mother to daughter to granddaughter; assists transmission of women's mysteries through the generations, carries forward the secrets of the Goddess and Her women, continues the rituals of the Goddess Craft; opens women's spiritual knowledge and psychic abilities; aids in Goddess rituals, Drawing Down the Moon, rites of passage, ritual connection with one's foremothers and the Goddess; symbolically heals the blood and the womb, promotes fertility

CHAIN OF LOVE
(Antigonon leptopus)
(Heart) Pink

Add Gemstones: Pink Coral, Pink Kunzite, Pink Tourmaline, Rhodonite, Pink Andean Opal, Pink Chinese Opal, Rose Quartz, Pink Smithsonite, Clear Quartz Crystal, Danburite

Attracts healthy love relationships especially for those who have not had healthy relationships in the past; assists being in relationship, developing new relationships, learning to live together; increases and promotes self-love and self-worth, increases self-validation and self-respect, promotes respect for one's partner, enhances harmony. Also called Mexican Love Chain.

CHENILLE PLANT
(Acalyphya hispida)
(Earth) Red

Add Gemstones: Garnet, Hematite, Obsidian, Healer's Gold, Black Tourmaline, Black Coral, Black Kyanite, Black Star Sapphire, Clear Quartz Crystal, Danburite

Promotes rootedness into this incarnation, develops and repairs the energetic grounding system (chakras, channels, cord, connections), connects the grounding cord properly into the core of the Earth; keeps one grounded and centered in all situations, promotes nurturance, makes one secure and stable; promotes focus upon one's life path and confidence in knowing one's life purpose; encourages knowing and respecting the Earth, offers help for planetary healers

CHINESE LANTERN
(Physalis heterophylla)
(Solar Plexus) Yellow

> **Add Gemstones:** Yellow Opal, Yellow Fluorite, Hessionite Garnet, Amber, Yellow Zincite, Yellow Kyanite, Lemon Yellow Calcite, Citrine, Herkimer Diamond, Danburite
>
> Increases and promotes perception of fairies, dryads, naiads and other nature devas; aids empathy and telepathy with domestic animals, wild animals, birds, reptiles, insects and plants; increases one's Earth awareness, helps those who work at clearing the land of past traumas, abuse and entities, good essence for planetary workers and healers; also a good essence to use in a sprayer for clearing gemstones

CHRISTMAS CACTUS
(Schlumbergera zygocactus)
(Heart) Pink

> **Add Gemstones:** Pink Tourmaline, Pink Sapphire, Watermelon Tourmaline, Pink Smithsonite, Pink Fluorite, Rose Quartz, Herkimer Diamond, Danburite

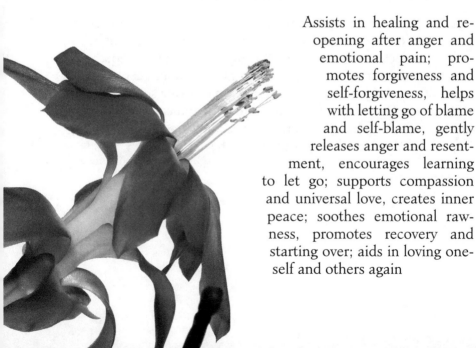

> Assists in healing and re-opening after anger and emotional pain; promotes forgiveness and self-forgiveness, helps with letting go of blame and self-blame, gently releases anger and resentment, encourages learning to let go; supports compassion and universal love, creates inner peace; soothes emotional rawness, promotes recovery and starting over; aids in loving oneself and others again

CHRISTMAS CACTUS
(Schlumbergera zygocactus)

(Root) Red

> **Add Gemstones:** Healers' Gold, Black Jade, Garnet, Red Coral, Ruby, Black Kyanite, Red Obsidian, Rainbow Obsidian, Black Opal, Clear Quartz Crystal, Danburite
>
> Supports healing and emotional reopening after a broken relationship, heals lost love, heals those who have been "dumped" by a lover; aids survivors of sexual abuse or battering; promotes emotional recovery and beginning a new relationship with new awareness, sustains new beginnings alone or with another lover; increases self-love, restores courage, regains strength and balance; provides protection in vulnerable times of change

CHRISTMAS CACTUS
(Schlumbergera zygocactus)

(Heart) White

> **Add Gemstones:** Chrysoprase, Emerald, Green Fluorite, Green Aventurine, Green Jade, Dioptase, Green Kunzite, Green Calcite, Herkimer Diamond, Danburite
>
> Assists in emotional reopening after grief, loss, hurt, trauma or disappointment; protects tenderness and vulnerability, cushions lost innocence; aids new starts and new beginnings in life; supports emotional recovery and convalescence, helps in regaining strength and hope; reduces shyness and fear, promotes courage, rebalances, offers emotional protection and buffering

CHRISTMAS PLANT
(Euphurbia sp.)

(Root) Red and Green

> **Add Gemstones:** Bloodstone, Green Jasper, Red Jasper, Pyrite, Green Onyx, True Jade, Serpentine Green Jade, Red Garnet, Hematite, Clear Quartz Crystal, Danburite
>
> Offers courage, inner strength, determination, grounding; can be used to stabilize kundalini energy reactions, grounds psychic opening, reduces psychic impressions if they become frightening or too distracting, gives a too-open psychic a temporary rest, stabilizes; a supportive energy for balancing the blood—for hemorrhaging, blood-building and blood disorders. Also called Florida Poincetta.

CLARODENDRUM
(Clarodendron speciosissimum)

(Root) Red

> **Add Gemstones:** Red Spinel, Garnet, Moroccan Red Quartz, Ruby, Star Ruby, Black Tourmaline, Black Kyanite, Hematite, Red Obsidian, Red Pietersite, Clear Quartz Crystal, Danburite
>
> Promotes balanced and responsible sexuality, helps those opening to sexuality for the first time; develops spiritual relationships, creates security in relationships; assists in rejecting abuse, helps with leaving abusive situations, helps to prevent and heal victimization. Also called Pagoda Flower.

CLEMATIS, Broughton Star

(Clematis sp.)

(Heart) Pink

Add Gemstones: Rhodochrosite, Gem Rose Quartz, Pink Calcite, Raspberry Garnet, Pink Tourmaline, Pink Andean Opal, Pink Coral, Herkimer Diamond, Danburite

Provides strong energy cleansing and purification of the hara and kundalini channels and chakras, clears obstructions especially of the heart complex chakras and channels; heals and opens the heart on all levels, ends being emotionally stuck; releases karmic obstructions and heart scars but may not do so gently, releases heart blocks originating in past lives and from negative karmic patterns of the heart and emotions; aids healing of this life past abuse; promotes emotional transformation, offers support for all emotional and heart healing

CLEMATIS, General Sikorski

(Clematis sp.)

(Third Eye) Dark Blue

Add Gemstones: Azurite, Blue Aventurine, Lapis Lazuli, Blue Chalcedony, Blue Pietersite, Sodalite, Blue Sapphire, Iolite, Celestite, Herkimer Diamond, Danburite

Strong energy cleansing properties for purification of the hara and kundalini line chakras and channels, clears obstructions, reduces and clears the inability to move forward in one's life, ends being stuck; promotes mental transformation and change, heals the mental body levels, promotes core soul healing; removes emotional attachments and negative thought forms, heals negative karmic patterns; aids and increases psychic development and evolution, increases insight

CLEMATIS, Ramona
(Clematis sp.)

(Throat) Light Blue

> **Add Gemstones:** Angelite, Blue Sapphire, Celestite, Azurite, Lapis Lazuli, Sodalite, Amazonite, Blue Lace Agate, Blue Andean Opal, Herkimer Diamond, Danburite
>
> Offers strong energy cleansing and purification of mental body chakras and the hara line and kundalini chakras and channels; especially clears obstructions of the throat complex and third eye, opens the throat chakras on the mental body level; removes karmic throat blockages, removes blocks to one's ability to speak out or speak one's mind or needs; aids all creativity, especially helps singers and speakers, opens the throat on all levels, increases psychic ability

CLEMATIS, Red Cardinal
(Clematis sp.)

(Earth) Dark Red

> **Add Gemstones:** Red Garnet, Ruby, Black Star Sapphire, Black Kyanite, Black Tourmaline, Obsidian, Black Quartz, Tektite, Clear Quartz Crystal, Danburite
>
> Provides strong energy cleansing and purification of the hara and kundalini channels and chakras, clears obstructions; reduces and clears the inability to move forward on one's earthly path, ends being stuck; connects one's spiritual life purpose with earth plane action and competence, removes indecisiveness and uncertainty; aids earth plane-oriented change and transformation; heals fear, clears and heals the etheric body for physical healing, strengthens one's connection and grounding to the planet

CLOVER, Red
(Trifolium sp.)
(Causal Body) Red

Add Gemstones: Watermelon Tourmaline, Pink Tourmaline, Red Garnet, Raspberry Garnet, Ruby, Star Ruby, Ruby with Zoisite, Clear Quartz Crystal, Danburite

Cleanses, clears and repairs the emotional body; aligns, clears and repairs the hara line chakras; develops and opens the causal body chakra; promotes reception of psychic information, promotes automatic writing and channeling, stabilizes mediums; increases connection with angels, spirit guides, Lords of Karma, star guides, Goddess and the Light; spiritualizes one's life and life purpose; helps in giving and receiving unconditional love, aids forgiveness of oneself and others, helps in knowing Goddess

CLOVER, White
(Trifolium sp.)
(Vision) White

Add Gemstones: Aragonite, Phantom Quartz, Seer Stone, Clear Fluorite, Clear Beryl, Clear Kunzite, Clear Calcite, White Sapphire, Selenite, Phenacite, Herkimer Diamond, Danburite

Insists upon one's seeing what must be seen; opens visions of old traumas from this and past lives so they can be faced and released, assists in opening and releasing; removes karmic blocks, releases karmic patterns to be faced and healed; opens the veils to reveal what has been hidden; increases all psychic abilities—clairvoyance, mediumship, crystal gazing, channeling, prophecy; sometimes causes visions of future lifetimes, does not always work gently

CONEFLOWER, Fragrant Angel
(Echincea purpurea)

(Crown) White

> **Add Gemstones:** Diamond, Clear Beryl, Clear Kunzite, White Moonstone, Snow Quartz, White Apophyllite, Rainbow Moonstone, Phenacite, Herkimer Diamond, Danburite

> Supports innocence and childhood, an essence for babies and small children; helps in adjusting to physical form, helps in learning and growing without fear; protects the crown chakra in small children, protects children's ability to go in and out of body when very small; offers connection to protecting and teaching angels, enhances understanding and communication with the angelic realm, supports children's ability to remain spiritual Be-ings although in physical form, helps children remember who they really are as spiritual Be-ings; enhances children's connection with Goddess. Also known as Echinacea, the all-healing herb.

CONEFLOWER, Green Envy
(Echinacea purpurea)

(Diaphragm) Green

> **Add Gemstones:** Yellow Zincite, Green Tourmaline, Malachite, Yellow Apatite, Yellow Jade, Green Jade, Green Garnet, Peridot, Golden Beryl, Emerald, Herkimer Diamond, Danburite

> Cleanses the hara line and emotional body of toxic emotions; makes one realize the karma of envy, jealousy and greed; can show past life pictures of toxic emotional situations and their damage; reveals karmic patterns from past lifetimes regarding hate, malice and other negativity; helps in releasing and ending negative emotions from this and past lifetimes and aids in ending harmful karmic patterns; changes negativity to acceptance and forgiveness, ends blame and vengeance; not always a gentle essence or lesson. Also called Echinacea, the all-healing herb.

CONEFLOWER, Pink Double Delight
(Echinacea purpurea)
(Heart) Pink

Add Gemstones: Raspberry Garnet, Rubellite (Pink Tourmaline), Pink Sapphire, Pink Calcite, Pink Kunzite, Pink Coral, Lazurine, Herkimer Diamond, Danburite

Brings joy and delight, childlike innocence, heals the heart; cleanses, clears and repairs the heart chakra, heart complex and emotional body; restores the joy that has been lost to lifetimes of suffering and damage; promotes the will to live, increases enjoyment and eagerness, changes apathy to curiosity, changes anger into forgiveness and acceptance; releases the karma of suffering and grief left from past lifetimes, prevents suffering and trauma from this lifetime from becoming karmic; restores inner peace. Also known as Echinacea, an all-healing herb.

CONEFLOWER, Vintage Wine
(Echinacea purpurea)
(Root) Red

Add Gemstones: Ruby, Star Ruby, Garnet, Red Spinel, Red Coral, Moroccan Red Quartz, Red Phantom Quartz, Clear Quartz Crystal, Danburite

Warms and makes one feel wanted, promotes feeling cared about and needed in this world, promotes feeling that one has a place here; increases the flow of life force (Light or ch'i) into the kundalini line, repairs and opens the root chakra and kundalini channels; stabilizes and grounds while freeing one to reach out and astral travel safely; enhances the will to live, increases love of living, inspires the need and ability to explore and grow; brings the spirit fully into the physical body, spiritualizes the physical Be-ing. Also called Echinacea, the all-healing herb.

COREOPSIS
(Coreopsis grandiflora)

(Solar Plexus) Yellow

Add Gemstones: Yellow Jade, Golden Calcite, Natural Citrine, Amber, Yellow Fluorite, Yellow Kyanite, Yellow Opal, Herkimer Diamond, Danburite

Increases psychic ability and psychic strength, brings in and assimilates psychic information; promotes understanding of psychic information, psychic vision, clairvoyance, inner knowing; promotes putting psychic input into perspective with physical reality; good aid to studying (spiritual or earthly)

CORN
(Zea mays)

(Solar Plexus) Yellow

Add Gemstones: Yellow Opal, Golden Topaz, Yellow Fluorite, Natural Citrine, Yellow Kyanite, Yellow Sunstone, Golden Calcite, Herkimer Diamond, Danburite

Promotes physical and spiritual nourishment, material and inner security; increases prosperity, enhances physical and spiritual fulfillment, promotes success, increases spiritual wealth (the inner things that matter) and provides well-being; fosters inner peace, brings the Goddess into one's life; the Native American Mother of Life. Corn is a symbol of riches and wealth in the Victorian language of flowers.

COSMOS
(Cosmos bipinnatus)
(Thymus) Multi Colors

Add Gemstones: Turquoise, Aquamarine, Clear Beryl, Clear Topaz, Emerald, Morganite, Clear Quartz Crystal, Danburite

Promotes honoring the oneness of all life; provides a sense of blessing to oneself and others, aids giving and receiving in balance, increases generosity, promotes harmony in groups; aids the ability to forgive others and oneself, heals guilt and blame, heals self-blame, changes grief to joy; aids animal communication

CRAPE MYRTLE
(Lagerstroemia indica)
(Crown) Lavender

Add Gemstones: Amethyst, Sugilite, Holly Blue Agate, Purple Fluorite, Pink Tourmaline, Lepidolite, Violet Tourmaline, Clear Quartz Crystal, Danburite

Creates a union of intellect and emotion; promotes without sadness the qualities of calmness, steadiness, responsibility, sobriety, carefulness, spirituality and devotion; aids in self-acceptance, positive self-validation, unconditional love for oneself and others; good support for those learning to meditate or beginning and opening to spiritual study

CRAPE MYRTLE
(Lagerstroemia indica)

(Heart) Pink

> **Add Gemstones:** Pink Kunzite, Rose Quartz, Pink Tourmaline, Pink Jade, Pink Andean Opal, Pink Garnet, Pink Sapphire, Clear Quartz Crystal, Danburite
>
> Promotes repair and healing of the emotional body from all damage and injury, including karmic damage brought from other lifetimes; provides heart healing, brings love into one's life; encourages positive self-love, aids in forgiveness of oneself and others, establishes the beginnings of unconditional love; enables joy in living, increases trust and openness, soothes and calms

CRAPE MYRTLE
(Lagerstroemia indica)

(Perineum) Red

> **Add Gemstones:** Ruby with Zoisite, Ruby, Garnet, Red Siberian Quartz, Moroccan Red Quartz, Snow Quartz, White Moonstone, Phenacite, Herkimer Diamond, Danburite
>
> Manifests love on the earth plane; helps in finding and recognizing one's soul mate, aids in starting and developing a soul mate relationship; makes physical relationships both physical and spiritual, supports the union of souls and bodies, helps in sustaining long term marriages and loving relationships; helps in opening to receive love of all kinds, promotes unconditional love for others and oneself

CRAPE MYRTLE
(Lagerstroemia indica)

(Transpersonal Point) White

Add Gemstones: White Moonstone, Peach Moonstone, White Calcite, Phenacite, Selenite, Snow Quartz, Diamond, Rutile Quartz, Clear Quartz Crystal, Danburite

Promotes marriage or union for life and beyond, buffers the difficulties of sustaining a long term union; promotes fidelity, truth and trust in relationships; develops and sustains soul bonding between lovers, promotes love that is total and eternal, promotes unconditional love for each other; brings together and keeps together karmic soul mates and twin souls, helps to sustain eternal love

CROCUS, Dutch

(Crown) Deep purple

Add Gemstones: Amethyst, Amethyst with Hematite, Rutile Amethyst, Purple Sapphire, Violet Tourmaline, Purple Obsidian, Herkimer Diamond, Danburite

For remembrance, heals the past in this life and from past incarnations; heals karmic patterns, releases karma, heals this lifetime by promoting understanding of one's past lifetimes; aids the death transition, helps those on the path of spiritual growth, promotes and accelerates enlightenment (ascension)

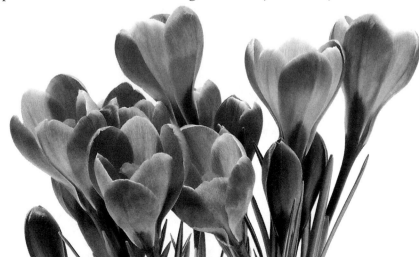

CROCUS, Golden
(Crocus chrysanthus)
(Solar Plexus) Yellow

Add Gemstones: Golden Calcite, Natural Citrine, Golden Amber, Yellow Opal, Yellow Topaz, Yellow Jade, Yellow Fluorite, Clear Quartz Crystal, Danburite

For karmic healing, promotes joy in being alive, offers a new life with a new perspective on life, releases karmic patterns that prevent a joyful life, heals karmic suffering; good essence for infants and small children who seem troubled or unhappy to be here, offers hope. Traditional Victorian flower symbol for mirth.

CROCUS, Scotch
(Crocus biflorus)
(Crown) Pale lavender

Add Gemstones: Lepidolite, Lepidolite with Rubellite, Kyanite with Rubellite, Amethyst, Violet Tourmaline, Sugilite, Charoite, Herkimer Diamond, Danburite

Encourages interest in spirituality, enhances spiritual growth, initiates psychic development and opening; helps in learning to use one's psychic abilities, aids learning to not be afraid of psychic happenings; encourages understanding oneself as a spiritual Be-ing, promotes past life recall and working with the Lords of Karma; initiates connection with Goddess and the Light

CROCUS, Snow
(Crocus chrysanthus)
(Crown) White

> **Add Gemstones:** Phenacite, Snow Quartz, White Opal, Fire Opal, White Druzy Quartz, Phantom Quartz, White Calcite, Phantom Calcite, Clear Quartz Crystal, Danburite
>
> For accessing and understanding past lives and past life patterns; helps with the beginnings of karmic understanding, aids karmic release, promotes understanding death and rebirth, promotes knowing that we have been here before, aids in learning one's own karmic herstory; provides contact one's own and others karmic records (the Akashic Records) for karmic healing and release; promotes working with the Lords of Karma

CROSSANDRA
(Crossandra infundibuliformis)
(Hara) Orange

> **Add Gemstones:** Orange Sunstone, Yellow Sunstone, Peach Moonstone, White Moonstone, Orange Calcite, Carnelian, Herkimer Diamond, Danburite
>
> For opening and expanding all psychic abilities—especially clairvoyance, psychic healing, clairaudience, channeling; increases communication with spirit guides and angels, brings in increased Light energy, supports new psychics and beginning channelers, promotes self-confidence in one's abilities and in the psychic realm; protects psychics from negative interference

DAHLIA, Black Diamond
(Dahlia sp.)

(Earth) Red-Black

> **Add Gemstones:** Black Tourmaline, Black Obsidian, Rainbow Obsidian, Tektite, Hematite, Amethyst with Hematite, Diamond, Clear Quartz Crystal, Danburite
>
> For connection with the planet and physical form; promotes Earth stewardship and aids those who help and heal the planet, encourages being an Earth advocate, supports those who walk softly on the Mother; aids all environmental efforts and activism, aids those who help the animals (all kinds, domestic and wild) and other planet life forms (insects, reptiles, birds, etc.); protects activists and planetary healers from others' malice and interference; helps activists and healers to see the results of their efforts, helps to prevent and heal burnout and despair

DAHLIA, Caliente
(Dahlia sp.)

(Perineum) Red

> **Add Gemstones:** Spinel, Red Garnet, Ruby, Amethyst with Hematite, Hematite, Red Moroccan Quartz, Bulico Jasper, Red Jasper, Clear Quartz Crystal, Danburite
>
> Connects the hara line and kundalini line channels at the root; increases energy flow and movement, increases energy levels, brings in increased life force energy (ch'i) from above and below; strengthens energy flow that comes through the root chakra from the Earth, promotes stability and determination; strengthens energy flow from the Light that enters through the crown, helps to spiritualize daily life; promotes joy, fosters passion for living and sexual passion, encourages physical and earth plane love that is also spiritual love

DAHLIA, Peggy Jean
(Dahlia sp.)

(Solar Plexus) Yellow

Add Gemstones: Lemon Yellow Calcite, Citrine, Rutile Citrine, Yellow Fluorite, Golden Topaz, Golden Beryl, Golden Labradorite, Clear Quartz Crystal, Danburite

Fills the aura and kundalini chakras with Light and peace; heals and repairs rips, tears and holes in the aura and auric field; aligns and balances the kundalini line chakras and channels, cleanses and clears, removes obstructions and blockages, ends most interference; clears released karma and karmic artifacts from the aura and chakras but does not offer karmic release in itself; promotes clarity on all levels especially mental clarity, provides a clear mind, reduces confusion and chatter

DAHLIA, Purple Taiheijo
(Dahlia sp.)

(Crown) Purple

Add Gemstones: Purple Spirit Quartz, Amethyst, Canadian Amethyst, Amethyst Quartz Charoite, Sugilite, Violet Tourmaline, Lepidolite, Herkimer Diamond, Danburite

Enhances and increases spiritual growth and evolution, promotes the path to enlightenment or ascension, assists incarnated Bodhisattvas and those on the Bodhisattva Path; helps those in service to the planet and people, strengthens healers and teachers; promotes psychic opening and development; reduces stress, burnout, exhaustion, overwhelm, despair, insomnia, nightmares; calms, soothes and heals

DAHLIA, Victoria Ann
(Dahlia sp.)
(Crown) Lavender and White

> **Add Gemstones:** Purple Kunzite, Pink Sapphire, Purple Sapphire, Violet Tourmaline, Lepidolite, Charoite, Amethyst, Sugilite, Herkimer Diamond, Danburite
>
> For gentle opening to channeling and other psychic skills; initiates and accelerates spirituality and spiritual evolution; promotes all evolutionary paths (enlightenment, ascension) and all soul growth; brings one into contact with Goddess and the Light, increases contact and communication with all Light Be-ings, promotes angelic contact and contact with the Lords of Karma; makes every aspect of psychic and spiritual awakening safe and gentle, promotes security and comfort, ends fear of spiritual opening and psychic contact, balances kundalini rising incidents; heals and repairs the crown chakra

DAISY, Gerber
— *See GERBER DAISY*

DAISY, Shasta
(Leucanthemum x superbum)
(Crown) White

> **Add Gemstones:** Clear Beryl, White Topaz, Clear Fluorite, Selenite, Snow Quartz, Phenacite, White Calcite, Clear Quartz Crystal, Danburite
>
> For regaining lost innocence, aids in restoring trust after betrayal and loss; helps to heal traumatic loss, assists grief recovery; aids regaining emotional equilibrium, restores mental rebalancing after shock or traumatic grief, aids those surviving loss or disaster or all kinds; promotes emotional rescue in emergencies and stress

DAISY, Wild
(Bellis perennis)
(Crown) White

Add Gemstones: Pink Kunzite, Pink Tourmaline, Watermelon Tourmaline, Rose Quartz, Pink Calcite, Green Calcite, Green Aventurine, Clear Quartz Crystal, Danburite

Protects the innocence of children and of adults who wish to retain or regain their child-like innocence; promotes gentleness of thoughts and actions, is a buffer against the pressures of modern life; aids keeping one's innocence and purity in a cynical world; acts as an emotional shield, offers emotional protection, purifies, soothes

DANDELION
(Taraxacum officinale)
(Diaphragm) Yellow

Add Gemstones: Natural Citrine, Peridot, Amber Calcite, Yellow Fluorite, Yellow Opal, Green Amber, Golden Amber, Yellow Jade, Herkimer Diamond, Danburite

Cleanses and purifies the physical, emotional and mental bodies; releases old emotions from this life and past lifetimes, heals the past and promotes moving forward, releases being stuck in past hurts; balances and increases energy flows in the kundalini and hara energy systems, enhances the intellect and all mental processes, brings in the Light to illuminate all darkness, eases resentment and fear

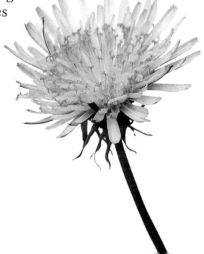

DAYLILY, Crimson Pirate
(Hemerocallis sp.)

(Belly) Orange

> **Add Gemstones:** Red Jasper, Mookite, Mexican Opal, Orange Zincite, Orange Calcite, Red-Orange Agate, Carnelian, Clear Quartz Crystal, Danburite
>
> Supports emotional growth and sustenance, promotes harvesting what one has sown; enhances the stability and fulfillment of one's life purpose, aids in finding and recognizing one's life purpose, stimulates the desire to follow one's life path, provides emotional and physical rewards for hard work done well; stimulates the life force and the will to live, promotes emotional survival, heals grief

DAYLILY, Miniature
(Hemerocallis sp.)

(Solar Plexus) Gold and Red

> **Add Gemstones:** Natural Citrine, Red Jasper, Yellow Jasper, Mookite, Mexican Opal, Yellow Opal, Yellow Jade, Amber, Clear Quartz Crystal, Danburite
>
> Facilitates energy replenishment on physical, emotional, mental and spiritual body levels; helps burnout, exhaustion, debility; supports recovery from trauma, traumatic stress, mental stress, illness, surgery, childbirth, overexertion, overexposure to cold or heat; provides stabilization and stability, promotes a feeling of well-being, offers calm energy enhancement, provides extra endurance without nervousness

DELPHINIUM
— See LARKSPUR

DIANTHUS, Desmond
(Dianthus desmond)

(Root) Red

Add Gemstones: Cuprite, Amethyst with Hematite, Ruby, Red Obsidian, Red Moroccan Quartz, Garnet, Clear Quartz Crystal, Danburite

Turns sexual passion into spiritual love, turns a fling into a relationship, turns a relationship into a marriage; brings joy and delight into one's sexuality along with caring and respect for the other person; makes sex without love distasteful, makes sex with love fulfilling and spiritual; promotes deep caring and real love, promotes true love; helps to establish new relationships and turn them into long term unions, supports enduring love and fulfilling passion in long term relationships; balances and heals the root chakra

DIANTHUS, Sweet William
(Dianthus barbatus)

(Heart) Pink and Purple

Add Gemstones: Stichtite, Pink Kunzite, Purple Kunzite, Amethyst, Violet Tourmaline, Pink Tourmaline, Lepidolite, Cobaltite, Pink Calcite, Clear Quartz Crystal, Danburite

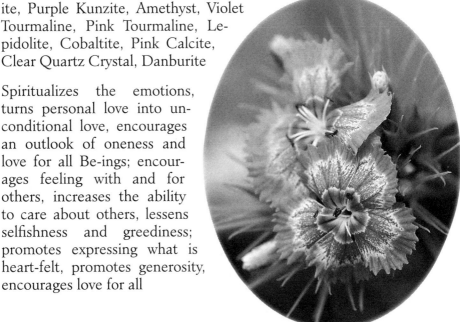

Spiritualizes the emotions, turns personal love into unconditional love, encourages an outlook of oneness and love for all Be-ings; encourages feeling with and for others, increases the ability to care about others, lessens selfishness and greediness; promotes expressing what is heart-felt, promotes generosity, encourages love for all

DIPLADENIA
(Dipladenia splendens)
(Heart) Pink and Yellow

> **Add Gemstones:** Pink Druzy Quartz, Rhodonite, Pink Chinese Opal, Cobaltite, Rose Quartz, Pink Sapphire, Pink Tourmaline, Kunzite, Herkimer Diamond, Danburite

> Turns suffering into joy, encourages letting go of the thought that life has to be hard, releases suffering from one's karmic blueprint; allows joy to enter and become one's life, ends the thought that happiness is only for others; promotes letting go of despair, anguish, karmic guilt, shame and self-blame; offers the ability to receive joy and be happy

DWARF POINCIANA
— *See POINCIANA, Dwarf*

ECHINACEA
— *See CONEFLOWER*

ESPERANZA
(Tecoma stans)
(Diaphragm) Yellow

> **Add Gemstones:** Yellow Kyanite, Amber, Yellow Opal, Yellow Fluorite, Golden Labradorite, Tiger Eye, Yellow Jade, Clear Quartz Crystal, Danburite

> Cleanses, clears and detoxifies the hara line and emotional body; helps those who lack the will to live, increases interest in one's life and in how one lives it, encourages a sense of pride and purpose; stimulates a sense of wellness and well-being, of being in the right place at the right time; increases hope, heals apathy, raises moods, brings in joy and Light, promotes starting new friendships; removes negative interference and offers psychic protection

FALSE HIBISCUS
(Malviavuscus arboreus)
(Root) Red

Add Gemstones: Red Spinel, Ruby, Garnet, Moroccan Red Quartz, Healers' Gold, Pyrite, Black Kyanite, Red Obsidian, Herkimer Diamond, Danburite

Promotes living fully in the body and on the earth plane; encourages knowing truth from falsehood, separates reality from illusion, develops discernment; promotes being truthful and honest, encourages integrity; inspires taking care and having competence in daily life, fosters making an honest living, promotes being responsible in one's actions and deeds, increases having good intention in all things; aids in being grounded and centered without heaviness or feeling tied down. Also called Turkish Hats; the flowers resemble the fez.

FLAME VINE
(Pyrostegiaignea)
(Belly) Orange

Add Gemstones: Pecos Quartz, Carnelian, Mexican Opal, Red Jasper, Moroccan Red Quartz, Spinel, Garnet, Clear Quartz Crystal, Danburite

Attracts and stimulates sexual love; increases sexual attraction between lovers, assists courtship, aids in all aspects of sexuality; increases orgasm, increases fertility and conception if sex is unprotected; strives for physical and spiritual union between lovers but focuses on the physical and sexual

FLORIDA HONEYSUCKLE
(Bignonia)

(Belly) Orange

> **Add Gemstones:** Orange Calcite, Poppy Carnelian, Fuchsite, Jacinth (Orange Sapphire), Peach Moonstone, Sunstone, Peach Aventurine, Herkimer Diamond, Danburite
>
> Heals painful memories and traumas from this lifetime, releases and clears emotional pain, supports the healing of body pain; helps in reducing fear, prevents nightmares, reduces or stops panic; restores sweetness to one's life, encourages hope and raises the possibility of joy and healing; frees one from the burden of ongoing emotional pain, restores a gentler life, promotes looking forward instead of back

FLOSS-SILK TREE
(Chorisia speciosa)

(Heart) Pink

> **Add Gemstones:** Gem Rose Quartz, Pink Fluorite, Lepidolite, Kunzite, Pink Jade, Pink Andean Opal, Moonstone, Herkimer Diamond, Danburite
>
> Heals and repairs the emotional body on all levels, heals and repairs the heart chakra and heart complex (heart chakra on all levels); heals one's relationships with oneself and others, aids in learning to be cooperative with others in love affairs and in community situations, promotes learning to live together with a lover or mate; enhances positive self love, promotes holding love in one's heart at all times, inspires unconditional love

FORSYTHIA
(Forsythia lynwood)
(Solar Plexus) Yellow

> **Add Gemstones:** Peridot, Chrysoprase, Natural Citrine, Lemon Yellow Calcite, Yellow Sunstone, Yellow Fluorite, Serpentine Jade, Yellow Jade, Clear Quartz Crystal, Danburite
>
> An essence for prosperity and success, promotes abundance of all kinds (monetary, material, emotional); increases one's ability to receive, increases one's ability to manifest goodness; heals greed, envy and jealousy, insecurity, miserliness; promotes balance in spending and good money management, increases one's ability to save money; supports responsible shopping, increases generosity, balances giving and receiving, balances spending for oneself and giving to others

FOXGLOVE, Pam's Choice
(Crown) White and Maroon

> **Add Gemstones:** Lepidolite, Lepidolite with Mica, Charoite, Pink Tourmaline, Purple Kunzite, Sugilite, Selenite, Herkimer Diamond, Danburite
>
> Opens and clears the crown chakra, repairs crown damage; promotes, aids and stabilizes spiritual evolution--the ascension/enlightenment process; aids angelic contact, promotes contact with the Goddess, Lords of Karma, and one's spirit guides; promotes karmic clearing and release, enhances ones' trust in the Light and the process of soul evolution; calms and comforts, fills the energy channels with Light and healing

FRANGIPANI
(Plumeria rubra)

(Heart) Pink

> **Add Gemstones:** Morganite, Pink Calcite, Pink Lazurine, Lepidolite, Pink Tourmaline, Petalite, Rhodochrosite, Pink Sapphire, Clear Quartz Crystal, Danburite
>
> Balances and heals the female heart, heals the heart chakra and heart complex (all the heart levels), heals and comforts the emotions and emotional body; promotes positive self-image, makes one emotionally independent, aids in learning to take care of oneself and take charge of one's life; increases self-respect in relationships; helps to heal past emotional abuse, helps in emotional trauma recovery; heals body image, assists and supports those who are overcoming addictions

FRANGIPANI
(Plumeria rubra)

(Root) Red

> **Add Gemstones:** Canadian Amethyst, Garnet, Ruby, Star Ruby, Rutile Amethyst, Moroccan Red Quartz, Red Calcite, Red Pietersite, Clear Quartz Crystal, Danburite
>
> Increases female active energy, balances action with receptivity, promotes assertiveness without aggression; eases shyness, eases the fear of expressing one's needs; balances yin and yang in women; helps in expressing anger safely, releases anger; develops courage, increases the life force and will to live, heals and repairs the root chakra

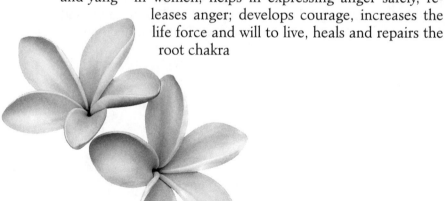

FRANGIPANI
(Plumeria rubra)
(Crown) White

Add Gemstones: White Moonstone, Fresh Water Pearl, Rainbow Moonstone, Phenacite, Snow Quartz, Clear Beryl, Clear Topaz, Clear Kunzite, Clear Quartz Crystal, Danburite

Increases female receptive energy, reduces and balances over-action and over-reaction; calms aggressiveness, aids in asserting one's needs calmly, reduces nervousness, develops courage, promotes ability to express anger safely; increases stability and gentleness, promotes feeling secure and safe; increases yin in women, increases the life force

FRANGIPANI
(Plumeria rubra)
(Solar Plexus) Yellow

Add Gemstones: Citrine, Ametrine, Amber, Lemon Yellow Calcite, Yellow Topaz, Dravite (Golden Tourmaline), Golden Beryl, Golden Labradorite, Herkimer Diamond, Danburite

Promotes mental balance especially in women; heals the mental body and mind grid (higher level of the mental body) and mental level chakras, initiates core soul healing; supports mental health and stability, increases self-respect; promotes success in the material world, assists in job and vocational success, assists in success in business, increases prosperity and abundance; supports assimilation of energy on all levels

FRANGIPANI
(Plumeria rubra Puu Kahea)
(Root) Yellow and Red

> **Add Gemstones:** Moroccan Red Quartz, Garnet, Citrine, Yellow Sapphire, Mookite, Yellow Jasper, Red Jasper, Zincite, Clear Quartz Crystal, Danburite

> Balances women's sexuality on kundalini and hara line levels and above; focuses especially on the root, belly, and solar plexus chakras and chakra complexes; initiates core soul healing for these chakras; provides emotional healing and support for all women's sexuality concerns; aids recovery from sexual trauma, rape, incest, abuse, codependency, abortion; promotes good self-image, body image and self-esteem; encourages positive sexuality and sexual function, provides emotional support for healthy menstrual and reproductive system function; good remedy for girls at menarche who are unsure of their menses and their body and for women who have been abused

FREESIA
(Freesia variodos)
(All Aura) Mixed Colors

> **Add Gemstones:** Gem Rose Quartz, White Moonstone, Amber, Sponge Coral, Garnet, Turquoise, Iolite, Amethyst, Clear Quartz Crystal, Danburite

> Supports the entire aura and all the kundalini chakras; promotes love of life, increases one's joy in living and Be-ing; brings pleasure with each day, inspires an awareness of beauty in everything, fosters awareness of the oneness of all life; heals creativity and artistry of every sort, promotes craftsmanship; mood-raising, calming, lifts grief, reduces fear, helps to heal broken hearts

GARDENIA
(Gardenia jasminoides)
(Transpersonal Point) White

> **Add Gemstones:** Selenite, Chrysoprase, Green Aventurine, White Jade, Green Jade, Green Amber, Green Calcite, Clear Quartz Crystal, Danburite
>
> Promotes the creation of a Body of Light (Light Body) in those who are on the path of enlightenment or ascension; creates, heals, clears, opens the Light Body; promotes high level spiritual evolution in those ready to receive it, prepares those who wish to become ready for ascension; brings in and heals soul fragments and ends the karma of soul fragmentation and damage, promotes all core soul healing especially on the higher soul levels; repairs and connects the higher levels of DNA, merges the Light Body into the physical levels (brings the soul into the body); provides a fast track for spiritual growth of all kinds

GAZANIA, Talent Orange
(Gazania sp.)
(Belly) Orange

> **Add Gemstones:** Carnelian, Mexican Opal, Jelly Opal, Orange Calcite, Orange Sunstone, Amber, Red Aventurine, Clear Quartz Crystal, Danburite
>
> Stimulates and increases vitality and love of living; promotes joy, happiness, a satisfied mind, boundless energy; supports playfulness, loving sexuality, taking reasonable risks, independence, curiosity; aids learning new skills, increases study concentration; helps one to complete what they start, continues interest in a project through completion and after; helps in making one's avocation into one's vocation and gainful living

GERANIUM
(Geranium sp.)
(Heart) Pink

> **Add Gemstones:** Morganite, Cobaltite, Rhodochrosite, Pink Kunzite, Lepidolite, Watermelon Tourmaline, Pink Tourmaline, Clear Quartz Crystal, Danburite
>
> For becoming a priestess of the Goddess of Love (Ishtar, Venus, Aphrodite) figuratively or actually; promotes the ability to give and receive love, to be loving and a lover; also supports sensuality and sexuality, sexual excitement in relationships, orgasm and sexual play, fidelity and monogamy in established relationships, responsible conception or contraception; promotes building a stable and responsible marriage or union, also supports positive self-love

GERANIUM
(Geranium sp.)
(Root) Red

> **Add Gemstones:** Apache Tears Obsidian, Black Tektite, Red Coral, Garnet, Hematite, Amethyst with Hematite, Black Tourmaline, Red Tiger Eye, Clear Quartz Crystal, Danburite
>
> Stimulates passion for life and love, promotes wanting to be here, strengthens one's life force vitality; draws the right mate to you, supports maturity in love and relationships, aids in creating realistic and balanced relationships, promotes commitment and responsibility in marriage or long term relationships; aids sexual satisfaction with one's partner, aids in parenthood or the sharing of other creativity together; an essence for life and love

GERANIUM
(Geranium sp.)

(Transpersonal Point) White

> **Add Gemstones:** White Moonstone, Rainbow Moonstone, Selenite, White Opal, Snow Quartz, Phenacite, White Phantom Quartz, Clear Quaratz Crystal, Danburite
>
> For opening to spiritual awareness of the Goddess and the Goddess within; makes women aware of their connection to the Moon Goddess in Her many names, and to the moon and lunar cycles; enhances ritual work, priestessing and Drawing Down the Moon; promotes awakening spirituality and psychic ability, calms and stabilizes psychic and spiritual growth; creates a strong expansion and evolution of psychic ability and psychic energy; provides ritual and emotional support for women's moon cycles--ovulation, menstruation and menopause

GERBER DAISY
(Gerbera jamesonii)

(All Chakras)

Mixed Colors—Red, Orange, Yellow, Pink, Lavender, White

> **Add Gemstones:** Ruby, Garnet, Carnelian, Orange Calcite, Amber, Rose Quartz, Green Calcite, Amethyst, Snow Quartz, Clear Quartz Crystal, Danburite
>
> Balances the kundalini chakras, adjusts and opens the chakras, fills the kundalini line with Light and love; brings a sense of excitement about one's life, optimism, curiosity, enjoyment; promotes a feeling of security and hope, fosters anticipating one's days with delight; good essence for babies and children, good for adolescents

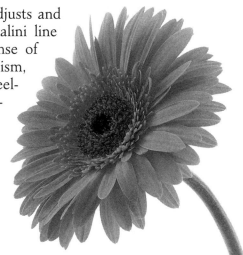

GERBER DAISY
(Gerber jamesonii)

(Belly) Orange

> **Add Gemstones:** Orange Calcite, Honey Calcite, Amber, Carnelian, Carnelian Agate, Vanadinite, Jacinth (Orange Sapphire), Mexican Opal, Clear Quartz Crystal, Danburite
>
> Balances and cleanses the belly chakra, releases old pictures of past hurts held in the chakra, flushes out old emotional grudges and resentments, cleanses the emotions and makes one free of the past; promotes moving forward in one's life, aids in preventing the past from corrupting the present, cleans the slate for a new beginning—if the person accepts it, initiates new beginnings and a brand new start

GERBER DAISY
(Gerber jamesonii)

(Heart) Pink

> **Add Gemstones:** Rose Quartz, Morganite, Pink Calcite, Pink Smithsonite, Pink Kunzite, Watermelon Tourmaline, Pink Tourmaline, Clear Quartz Crystal, Danburite
>
> Balances the mind with the emotions, the head with the heart; weighs "I want to" with "I should", makes one hesitate before jumping in; increases one's awareness of the consequences of one's actions; encourages choosing love but with awareness of one's mental reservations; promotes loving safely, promotes an open heart but a protected heart; encourages balance in all things

GERBER DAISY
(Gerber jamesonii)
(Root) Red

> **Add Gemstones:** Garnet, Spinel, Ruby, Pecos Quartz, Moroccan Red Quartz, Black Tourmaline, Obsidian, Amethyst with Hematite, Clear Quartz Crystal, Danburite
>
> Balances the root chakra, aligns the kundalini root with the hara line grounding chakras and channels; promotes balanced energy levels with stable grounding; increases emotional strength, promotes responsibility; stimulates the life force and the will to live; encourages passion in one's everyday life, balances sexual passion with caution, increases passion in love-making

GERBER DAISY
(Gerber jamesonii)
(Crown) White

> **Add Gemstones:** Snow Quartz, Clear Beryl, Clear Kunzite, Rainbow Moonstone, Phenacite, Optical Calcite, White Apophyllite, White Topaz, Clear Quartz Crystal, Danburite
>
> Protects and balances the crown chakra, clears the crown of blockages and obstructions, promotes opening the crown; increases and accelerates psychic and spiritual development gently, helps those who are afraid of spiritual opening; initiates first connection with Light Be-ings and Goddess, begins angelic contact, promotes connecting with one's spirit guides; enhances the ability to perceive and learn from spiritual guidance; starts one on the spiritual path

GERBER DAISY
(Gerber jamesonii)
(Solar Plexus) Yellow

> **Add Gemstones:** Lemon Yellow Calcite, Golden Beryl, Tiger Eye, Golden Labradorite, Amber, Yellow Fluorite, Natural Citrine, Rutile Citrine, Clear Quartz Crystal, Danburite
>
> Fills the kundalini line with Light and healing, balances and cleanses the solar plexus, heals damage to the solar plexus chakra; promotes mental clarity, aids concentration, increases effectiveness of study, aids memory and memorization, stops mental chatter, reduces flightiness; promotes new ideas, calms the mind

GINGER
(Hedychium Elizabeth)
(Heart) Pink

> **Add Gemstones:** Rhodochrosite, Gem Rose Quartz, Pink Tourmaline, Pink Jade, Pink Andean Opal, Rhodonite, Pink Kunzite, Herkimer Diamond, Danburite
>
> Heals the heart, heart complex (the heart system through all the levels), and emotional body; releases emotional heart scars from this and past lives gently; heals past emotional traumas, promotes the ability to trust again and to open one's heart, promotes the ability to give and receive love, enhances the knowing that you are loved; aids intimacy and the ability to give, warms the heart

GINGER, Bolivian Sunsex
(Curcuma sp.)
(Belly) Orange

> **Add Gemstones:** Orange Sunstone, Yellow Sunstone, Champagne Topaz, Orange Calcite, Jacinth (Orange Sapphire), Golden Selenite, Clear Quartz Crystal, Danburite
>
> Brings Light and healing into the womb, promotes sexual healing; emotional repair for sexual traumas—rape, incest, battering, sexual manipulation and abuse; heals negative birth (one's own birth) or giving birth experiences, provides emotional healing for the uterus and vagina; helps hysterectomy recovery; restores the ability to enjoy sex and appreciate one's body, increases orgasm

GINGER, Fiery Costus
(Costus cuspidatus)
(Belly) Orange

> **Add Gemstones:** Coral, Carnelian, Red-Orange Agate, Zincite, Vanadinite, Amber, Red Jade, Orange Garnet, Clear Quartz Crystal, Danburite
>
> Promotes orgasm, sexual opening, the giving and receiving of sexual pleasure, enhances sexual compatibility between partners, heals sexual shame and inhibition, encourages mutual joy and respect between sexual partners; helps women to become sexual again after abuse, rape or incest; promotes respect for the physical body, enhances positive body image, encourages self-esteem; encourages healthy and loving sexuality

GINGER, Shell
(Alpinia zerumbet)
(Heart) Pink and White

> **Add Gemstones:** Rose Quartz, Pink Calcite, Lepidolite, Pink Kunzite, Pink Tourmaline, Pink Sapphire, Cobaltite, Rhodochrosite, Clear Quartz Crystal, Danburite
>
> Warms the heart, promotes heart opening after emotional trauma and pain, facilitates emotional healing, aids grief recovery; heals past betrayal by a lover, releases old pain to encourage moving forward in one's life; regenerates and heals, promotes new joy, restores trust and hope, reduces stress and fear, aids in starting over

GINGER, Siam Tulip
(Curcuma alismatifolia)
(Heart and Root) Pink

> **Add Gemstones:** Pink Tourmaline, Watermelon Tourmaline, Raspberry Garnet, Raspberry Quartz, Pink Sapphire, Ruby, Star Ruby, Clear Quartz Crystal, Danburite
>
> Offers heart opening and sexual opening at once, promotes expression of true love via the sexual act; aids balanced sexuality, heals codependency, increases positive self-image and self-esteem; aids those who tend to confuse sex with real love, promotes developing real relationships in place of empty promiscuity; connects the root and heart chakras, removes obstructions and heals damage, heals the emotional body with regard to relationships and sexuality

GINGER, Sleeping Princess
(Curcuma sp.)

(Crown) White and Maroon

Add Gemstones: White Moonstone, Pink Tourmaline, Pink Chinese Opal, Lepidolite with Mica, Lepidolite with Rubellite, Rainbow Moonstone, Rhodonite, Sugilite, Clear Quartz Crystal, Danburite

Supports those who choose celibacy for spiritual purposes, aids spiritual opening and safe kundalini rising; supports astral (nonphysical) love and sex, and spiritual (physical and nonphysical) love unions; increases spiritual development and evolution, aids psychic development and soul growth, promotes one's connection with Goddess

GLADIOLUS, Alfalfa
(Gladiolus sp.)

(Causal body) Red-Violet

Add Gemstones: Raspberry Garnet, Pink Tourmaline, Cobaltite, Purple Kunzite, Pink Sapphire, Pink Druzy Quartz, Gem Rose Quartz, Gem Rhodochrosite, Herkimer Diamond, Danburite

Develops and opens the causal body chakra on the hara line, promotes psychic connection and reception of advanced spiritual Be-ings and advanced guidance; increases the level and amount of psychic information received and understood, increases the level of the Light Be-ings one can channel; promotes channeling, clairaudience (psychic hearing), automatic writing, karmic work, and empathy on a higher than third eye or kundalini throat chakra level; promotes accelerated psychic and spiritual development, accelerates all ascension (enlightenment) processes

GLADIOLUS, Blue Sky
(Gladiolus sp.)

(Third Eye) Blue

Add Gemstones: Azurite, Blue Aventurine, Blue Sapphire, Black Star Sapphire, Lapis Lazuli, Blue Pietersite, Blue Labradorite, Sodalite, Iolite, Blue Fluorite, Herkimer Diamond, Danburite

Promotes psychic visions and the ability to understand and use them; accelerates psychic opening and reception of psychic information; encourages clairvoyance, clairsentience, psychic healing, crystal gazing, visualization, clairaudience, telepathy, past life regression, future life progression, and other psychic skills; increases strength and frequency of psychic visions; increases contact with Light Be-ings, Goddess, spirit guides, angels, other-planetary healers; promotes spiritual transformation, accelerates spiritual growth and evolution

GLADIOLUS, Green Star
(Gladiolus sp.)

(Movement) Green

Add gemstones: Moldavite, Emerald, Green Tourmaline, Green Amber, Green Zincite, Epidote, Green Calcite, Green Garnet, Green Fluorite, Clear Quartz Crystal, Danburite

Initiates and encourages moving forward in one's life, ends being stuck, ends procrastination and resistance; soothes the way for those too afraid to take the next step, gives a harsher push to those who refuse to take the next step; causes an emotional detoxification and cleansing, brings out to be released old unsettled emotional issues and insists that they be looked at and resolved; purification, cleansing, energy clearing, releases blocks

GLADIOLUS, Tout a Toi
(Gladiolus sp.)

(Heart) Pink

> **Add Gemstones:** Rose Quartz, Gem Rose Quartz, Pink Tourmaline, Pink Calcite, Pink Fluorite, Moonstone, White Calcite, Clear Quartz Crystal, Danburite
>
> Brings gladness and joy into one's life, promotes and increases love of life and living, stabilizes the will to continue with one's life and life path; fosters the return of lost innocence, promotes appreciation of simple pleasures, returns joy after painful and hard times, aids and supports recovery from illness and debility; restores the ability to love and love again. Also called Sword Lily; the Victorian symbolism for this plant is strength of character

GLOXINIA
(Sinnimgia speciosa)

(Heart) Fuchsia

> **Add Gemstones:** Cobaltite, Pink Tourmaline, Rose Quartz, Pink Chinese Opal, Rhodochrosite, Pink Smithsonite, Clear Quartz Crystal, Danburite
>
> Brings love and universal love into the earth plane; supports the Earth changes by channeling love and healing onto the planet, promotes being a transmitter of love for planetary growth and change, promotes peace by holding and keeping peace in oneself; makes the concepts of self-love and love for others real; teaches unconditional love and forgiveness for oneself, others and the Earth

GLOXINIA
(Sinnimgia speciosa)
(Perineum) Maroon and White

> **Add Gemstones:** Garnet, Rutile Amethyst, Black Kyanite, Sugilite, Ruby, Star Ruby, Moroccan Red Quartz, Black Tourmaline, Clear Quartz Crystal, Danburite
>
> Connects the hara and kundalini line energy flows, connects the Earth and Sky, connects the Above and Below, and connects the root and crown; balances earth plane groundedness with spiritual purpose and awareness, promotes walking on Mother Earth as a spiritual Be-ing, helps Earth healers to remain stable and balanced while channeling psychic energy; grounds, centers, protects

GLOXINIA
(Sinnimgia speciosa)
(Vision) Purple and White

> **Add Gemstones:** Rutile Amethyst, Amethyst Quartz, Sugilite, Violet Tourmaline, Rainbow Moonstone, White Moonstone, Labradorite, Clear Fluorite, Danburite
>
> Stimulates psychic vision and out of body travel, aids seeing psychically for healing and Earth healing, increases the strength and range of distance psychic healing; helps with understanding and stabilization during the Earth changes, aids Earth healers and those helping souls to pass over; aids in holding and channeling psychic energy

GOLDEN CHALICE
(Solandra nitida zucs)

(Solar Plexus) Yellow

> **Add Gemstones:** Yellow Opal, Yellow Fluorite, Golden Topaz, Tiger Eye, Lemon Yellow Calcite, Yellow Jade, Clear Quartz Crystal, Danburite
>
> Stabilizes, calms and aids those who are dying; promotes acceptance and conscious dying, aids participation and cooperation with the death process; protects in the process and insures a peaceful transition, promotes awareness of guides and angels in the death process; promotes attaining enlightenment at the time of death, releases the soul from the body, reduces holding on in fear; provides rebalancing after a near death experience

GOLDEN SHOWERS TREE
(Cassia fistula)

(Solar Plexus) Yellow

> **Add Gemstones:** Pyrite, Emerald, Peridot, Natural Citrine, Golden Beryl, Yellow Opal, Yellow Jade, Green Jade, Clear Quartz Crystal, Danburite
>
> Draws and magnifies prosperity, increases abundance and success; promotes a sense of deserving the good things in life, increases the ability to receive, aids in manifesting; helps in balancing one's inner power, aids in finding a job you love, promotes good planning ability, increases good luck, brings "pennies from heaven"—unexpected money when most needed

GRAPEFRUIT BLOSSOM
(Citrus x paradisi)

(Third Eye) White

Add Gemstones: White Opal, Fire Opal, Chrysoprase, Green Turquoise, Green Aventurine, Green Jade, Serpentine Jade, Green Quartz, Green Kunzite, Herkimer Diamond, Danburite

Promotes balance, alignment and stability on physical and nonphysical levels; balances and aligns all the kundalini chakras and clears the channels, balances and aligns the energy bodies; repairs and rewires the energy systems, aids in regeneration of damaged energy systems, repairs the DNA; promotes clear thinking, calms and stabilizes, reduces stress

HEATHER
(Cuphea glutinosa)

(Crown) Purple

Add Gemstones: Lepidolite, Lepidolite with Mica, Sugilite, Amethyst, Purple Sapphire, Spirit Quartz, Purple Druzy Quartz, Herkimer Diamond, Danburite

Provides spiritual comfort and spiritual strength, offers the fortitude to face what must be faced no matter how difficult; eases anxiety and fear, reduces fear of dying or of pain, eases pain by increasing one's ability to relax and accept it, increases courage; eases inner or outward chatter, calms and increases faith, inspires trust; aids connection with spiritual guides and guidance

HIBISCUS
(Hibiscus rosa sinensis)

(All Aura) Multi Colors—One flower each of red, peach, yellow, rose and white

> **Add Gemstones:** Use all the colors: Garnet, Carnelian, Natural Citrine, Rose Quartz, Blue Calcite, Iolite, Amethyst, clear Quartz Crystal, Danburite

> Utilizes all the chakra colors to open and balance the entire kundalini system, stabilizes the physical body and lower nonphysical levels (the etheric and emotional levels); promotes spiritual growth and development, balances the energy systems, balances the physical with nonphysical levels; calms, an all-healing essence. The Victorians used this flower to designate delicate beauty.

HIBISCUS
(Hibiscus rosa sinensis)

(Belly) Peach

> **Add Gemstones:** Peach Moonstone, Champagne Topaz, Peach Calcite, Jelly Opal, Poppy Jasper, Pink Coral, Golden Beryl, Herkimer Diamond, Danburite

> An essence to support mothers and every aspect of pregnancy and motherhood; promotes fertility, conception, pregnancy, delivery, breast feeding; helps in adjusting emotionally to motherhood, bonding with infants, child rearing, resolving the problems of child raising and of being a mother, keeping one's identity as an independent adult while being a caretaker of small children; assists in finding wisdom, patience, energy, time, and joy in motherhood

HIBISCUS
(Hibiscus Rosa sinensis)

(Heart) Pink

> **Add Gemstones:** Morganite, Pink Druzy Quartz, Spirit Quartz, Pink Kunzite, Lepidolite, Rose Quartz, Pink Tourmaline, Watermelon Tourmaline, Clear Quartz Crystal, Danburite
>
> Heals betrayed trust and innocence, assists those in rape or incest recovery; heals heart hurts, betrayed relationships and friendships; helps those whose faith in life and the Goddess is broken, heals those with shattered trust; promotes core soul healing, assists in reintegrating shattered souls, brings in and heals soul fragments; heals the heart chakra and heart complex (heart on all levels); offers calm, hope and healing

HIBISCUS
(Hibiscus rosa sinensis)

(Root) Red

> **Add Gemstones:** Garnet, Spinel, Ruby, Black Tourmaline, Healer's Gold, Red Obsidian, Red Pietersite, Red Tiger Eye, Herkimer Diamond, Danburite
>
> Primarily for sexual healing; for healing and recovery from rape, battering, incest, all abuse; strengthens the life force, increases the will to live and prevail, helps all survival issues; offers emotional strength and spiritual protection; provides grounding and connection to the Earth and earth plane; promotes feeling secure and firmly in the body

HIBISCUS
(Hibiscus rosa sinensis)

(Transpersonal Point) White

> **Add Gemstones:** White Opal, Fire Opal, White Sapphire, White Moonstone, Rainbow Moonstone, Ulexite, White Calcite, Diamond, White Jade, Herkimer, Danburite
>
> Heals abandonment issues in children, adults, pets; promotes emotional recovery of all kinds, addiction recovery, recovery from battering, adult child recovery; supports self-determination, independence, self-reliance, empowerment, positive self-worth; assists those who must learn to live alone successfully and take care of their own needs; promotes an awareness of the oneness of all life, and of one's place in the universal plan

HIBISCUS
(Hibiscus rosa sinensis)

(Diaphragm) Yellow

> **Add Gemstones:** Yellow Sunstone, Natural Citrine, Golden beryl, Golden Labradorite, Amber, Yellow Topaz, Yellow Kyanite, Clear Quartz Crystal, Danburite
>
> Cleanses and purifies the aura and subtle bodies, releases and clears negative entities and attachments; heals tears in the aura and auric field, clears and expands the energy field and auric envelope; promotes a positive outlook and inner peace, aids gentle purification of all nonphysical levels and chakras, washes the aura, fills with Light

HOLLYHOCK
(Alcea rosa)

(Thymus) White

> **Add Gemstones:** Turquoise, Aquamarine, Gem Silica, Amazonite, Blue Andean Opal, Larimar, Aqua Kyanite, Blue Apatite, Herkimer Diamond, Danburite
>
> Heals and releases old grief and past sorrows that should have been long ago resolved, stops one from living in the past, moves one's life into the present, aids letting go of long-held pain and past hurts; releases despair, depression and hopelessness, replaces anger with acceptance, eases loneliness; finishes a stalled mourning process, promotes moving forward and going on

HONEYSUCKLE
(Lonicera semperevirens)

(Heart) Pink

> **Add Gemstones:** Pink Kunzite, Cobaltite, Pink Tourmaline, Lepidolite, Pink Sapphire, Rhodochrosite, Rhodonite, Herkimer Diamond, Danburite
>
> Facilitates contact and communication with fairies, dryads and devas, aids in seeing and perceiving nonphysical Be-ings and realms; brings childlike sweetness and joy into one's life, helps one to be gentle and loving with others, promotes innocence, gentleness and openness, provides emotional protection and security; protects dreams and dreamwork, calms and delights. Also see Florida Honeysuckle.

HYACINTH
(Hyacinthus orientalis)
(Causal Body) Blue

> **Add Gemstones:** Holly Blue Agate, Blue Chalcedony, Blue Quartz, Blue Kyanite, Blue Lace Agate, Blue Kyanite, Angelite, Iolite, Herkimer Diamond, Danburite
>
> Promotes conscious awareness of other dimensions, heals soul fragmentation and core soul damage; heals the Mind Grid, Earth Grid, and Galactic Grid energy structures, increases one's planetary and interplanetary awareness; aids in recognizing the needs of planet Earth; increases range of channeling and reception of information from spirit guides, angels and other-planetary helpers and healers; a good essence for channelers, psychic healers and Earth healers

HYACINTH
(Hyacinthus orientalis)
(Causal Body) Red

> **Add Gemstones:** Ruby, Star Ruby, Raspberry Garnet, Spinel, Moroccan Red Quartz, Cuprite, Rubellite, Kyanite, Kyanite with Rubellite, Herkimer Diamond, Danburite
>
> Stimulates becoming a consciously aware channel for Earth healing information received from other dimensions; initiates contact and communication with other-planetary and other-dimensional Light Be-ings; heals soul level damage in oneself and others via psychic healing; heals soul fragmentation, repairs DNA, helps in maintaining one's stability during Earth change energy shifts; opens positive intergalactic contact for oneself, other people, animals and the planet

HYACINTH
(Hyacinthus orientalis)
(Transpersonal Point) White

> **Add Gemstones:** White Moonstone, White Opal, Fire Opal, Selenite, White Fresh Water Pearl, Phenacite, Rainbow Moonstone, Snow Quartz, Herkimer Diamond, Danburite
>
> Channels other-dimensional help and healing into the four bodies (physical, emotional, mental, spiritual); promotes contact with healing and healers from other dimensions, realms and planets; opens and clears the kundalini and hara line chakras and energy flows, repairs and rewires the transpersonal point; repairs core soul damage, soul fragmentation, karmic damage, the DNA; aids spiritual evolution and enlightenment/ascension

HYACINTH, WATER
— *See WATER HYACINTH*

HYDRANGEA
(Hydrangea macrophylla)
(Throat) Blue

> **Add Gemstones:** Blue Mountain Jade, Blue Aventurine, Lapis Lazuli, Sodalite, Celestite, Angelite, Amazonite, Blue Opal, Blue Andean Opal, Larimar, Herkimer Diamond, Danburite
>
> For releasing what has long been unsaid, gets out what has been festering for needing expressed, releases and clears what has been emotionally stuck in one's throat; enhances the ability to speak one's personal truths, aids in expressing one's hurts and needs; heals relationships through positive honesty; heals anger, depression and rage by speaking out; promotes clearing and letting go of past traumas, hurts and pain by telling it aloud; ends the family secrets; helps and aids story telling, truth telling, speaking one's personal stories

HYDRANGEA
(Hydrangea macrophylla)

(Heart) Pink

Add Gemstones: Rhodochrosite, Rhodonite, Pink Druzy Quartz, Pink Tourmaline, Pink Kunzite, Purple Kunzite, Lepidolite, Herkimer Diamond, Danburite

Enhances the ability to speak out and say what is in one's heart, aids speaking from the heart with love, facilitates expressing emotions and feelings, aids the ability to express and demonstrate one's love for others; promotes positive self-love, establishes balanced assertiveness, makes it easier to take emotional risks

HYDRANGA
(Hydrangea macrophylla)

(Crown) Purple

Add Gemstones: Charoite, Spirit Quartz, Rutile Amethyst, Purple Fluorite, White Apophyllite, White Phantom Quartz, Selenite, Clear Quartz Crystal, Danburite

Promotes the ability to express spiritual truth and understanding in coherent thoughts and words, aids in understanding what one intuitively knows; aids in bringing spiritual intuition to concrete expression, adds logic to what one knows without words; makes the spiritual real and useful in everyday living, helps with finding the right word in daily situations; helps channelers, healers, writers, parents, teachers, artists

ICE PLANT, Mesa Verde
(Delosperma Mesa Verde)
(Heart) Pink

> **Add Gemstones:** Cobaltite, Lepidolite, Lepidolite with Rubellite, Pink Tourmaline, Raspberry Garnet, Gem Rose Quartz, Gem Rhodochrosite, Herkimer Diamond, Danburite
>
> Heals karmic damage to the kundalini heart chakra and the emotional body; brings old emotions from the emotional body to be released and healed, releases the karma of heartache and suffering that was not healed in the past lifetimes where it originated; dissolves and removes heart scars—may bring about revelations and karmic information with the release; lifts the weight of old karma from one's present life, promotes a healed heart; calms and soothes, provides release and relief

ICE PLANT, Red Mountain
(Delosperma dyeri cv. Psdold)
(Perineum) Red

> **Add Gemstones:** Garnet, Raspberry Garnet, Red Obsidian, Amethyst with Hematite, Spinel, Ruby, Star Ruby, Red Zincite, Herkimer Diamond, Danburite
>
> Promotes energy transformations of all kinds, increases the life force entering the physical and nonphysical bodies, brings in information from the planet core; provides intensive high energy levels with the ability to ground it and use it safely, uses the increased energy flows to bring about core soul healing; heals the emotional body, hara line, kundalini line, chakras and channels; balances the emotional with the physical, helps in accessing and releasing karma, provides the energy boost needed for spiritual acceleration

ICE PLANT, Starburst
(Delosperma floribundum)

(Crown) Purple

> **Add Gemstones:** Sugilite, Charoite, Amethyst, Rutile Amethyst, Violet Toumaline, Alexandrite, Purple Siberian Quartz, Clear Quartz Crystal, Danburite
>
> Promotes spiritual transformation; increases levels of spiritual energy entering all the nonphysical bodies and systems; initiates core soul healing and karmic healing on all levels, repairs and rewires the crown chakra and transpersonal point; releases karmic injury and damage, aids in doing conscious karmic release work with the Lords of Karma, promotes connection with the Lords of Karma; increases psychic opening, puts one on an accelerated spirituality path, pushes those reluctant to accept their psychic and spiritual abilities

IMPATIENS
(Impatiens sultanii)

(Transpersonal Point) White

> **Add Gemstones:** Oregon Opal (Opalite), Selenite, White Phantom Quartz, Moonstone, Snow Quartz, White Opal, Fire Opal, Rainbow Moonstone, Clear Quartz Crystal, Danburite
>
> An antidote for anger, haste, stress and worry by releasing one from the limits of time and the finite mind, promotes entering the bliss of the creational Void, aids in transcending the material and the earth plane; encourages spiritual awakening and spiritual evolution, offers an awareness of what is and is not important or real in life; aids in trusting the Goddess' nurturing and the Goddess' plan for one's life and for the All

IMPATIENS, Rosebud
(Impatiens, sp.)

(Heart) Fuchsia

> **Add Gemstones:** Pink Tourmaline, Cobaltite, Rose Quartz, Ruby, Ruby with Zoisite, Ruby with Fuchsite, Star Ruby, Pink Sapphire, Raspberry Garnet, Clear Quartz Crystal, Danburite
>
> Heals worry, stress, impatience; opens the heart to trusting life and the Goddess; makes it easier to flow with time and events, helps in understanding time as self-created by the mind, promotes living in the present gracefully and peacefully; aids in trusting the universe to provide means and opportunities, and aids in utilizing the opportunities offered; encourages trusting oneself and others, assists in knowing when to trust and when not to

IMPATIENS, Rosebud
(Impatiens, sp.)

(Root) Red

> **Add Gemstones:** Bloodstone, Ruby, Star Ruby, Red Spinel, Garnet, Canadian Amethyst, Amethyst with Hematite, Cuprite, Chalcotrichite, Clear Quartz Crystal, Danburite
>
> Supports the life force in times of dis-ease and weakness, helps debility and recovery from debility, reduces exhaustion, strengthens and heals; promotes patience in experiencing and waiting out an illness or dis-ease process; provides emotional support for surgical recovery, reduce worry and fear, stabilizes and calms

IRIS, Miniature Blue
(Iris reticulata)
(Third Eye) Blue

Add Gemstones: Blue Sapphire, Blue Kyanite, Lapis Lazuli, Azurite, Sodalite, Blue Aventurine, Holly Blue Agate, Phenacite, Herkimer Diamond, Danburite

Brings good fortune and the promise of a better future, heals the negative past from this and past lifetimes; clears the mind and mental body of negative thought forms and negative thinking patterns; provides the courage to heal and to change oneself for the better, offers emotional purification and mental growth, offers spiritual evolution; promotes awareness of the Goddess's blessings and Goddess within; increases and refines one's discernment, reduces stress and negative reactions to stress

IXORA
(Ixora coccinea)
(Belly) Peach

Add Gemstones: Peach Aventurine, Champagne Topaz, Peach Moonstone, Amber Calcite, Poppy Carnelian, Red Tiger Eye, Red Pietersite, Clear Quartz Crystal, Danburite

Cleanses the emotional and etheric bodies of old traumas by releasing flashbacks and pictures; also releases past life visions, aids past life regression and psychic visualization; removes negative cords and hooks from the Kundalini line; facilitates recovery from: incest, battering and rape, emotional and physical past abuse, old relationships, all trauma and traumatic incidents from this lifetime with possible flashbacks from past incarnations; uses the pictures stored in the belly chakra to reveal karmic patterns and release them. To focus on past lives and stimulate past life regression, use Phantom Quartz in the essence.

IXORA
(Ixora coccinea)

(Heart) Pink

> **Add Gemstones:** Pink Calcite, Cobaltite, Mangano Calcite, Rose Quartz, Pink Andean Opal, Pink Chinese Opal, Rhodonite, Herkimer Diamond, Danburite
>
> Clears the heart and emotional body of old traumas from this lifetime, releases heart scars from this life and past lives; heals emotional pain at the karmic source form this and past lives, ends karmic pain patterns; increases one's ability to give love to others and to receive it for oneself, aids opening to others emotionally, aids in making friends and being a friend; promotes learning to trust, reduces fear, soothes and calms

IXORA
(Ixora coccinea)

(Root) Red

> **Add Gemstones:** Bloodstone, Rainbow Obsidian, Red Obsidian, Black Tourmaline, Emerald, Red Jasper, Green Jasper, Fancy Jasper, Clear Quartz Crystal, Danburite
>
> Cleanses and purifies the kundalini line, cleanses the grounding system and root chakra; repairs the root chakra, releases and heals karmic damage to the root; supports those using holistic physical healing methods for blood and body cleansing, aids spiritual detoxification and purification processes; promotes development of healthy sexual boundaries, aids sexual healing

IXORA
(Ixora coccinea)
(Solar Plexus) Yellow

Add Gemstones: Natural Citrine, Golden Topaz, Golden Labradorite, Golden Fluorite, Yellow Kyanite, Golden Beryl, Amber, Herkimer Diamond, Danburite

Balances the Ch'i Kung and acupuncture meridian systems, opens blockages in meridian channels and acupuncture points to free energy flows and movement, opens and heals the hara line and aura body; provides mental cleansing, clears the mental body, aids the intellect and intellectual work of all kinds, balances energy levels throughout the mental and physical systems; heals exhaustion and depression, reduces burnout, promotes a positive outlook

JACARANDA TREE
(Jacaranda acutifolia)
(Crown) Purple

Add Gemstones: Sugilite, Canadian Amethyst, Brazilian Amethyst, Holly Blue Agate, Lepidolite, Lepidolite with Mica, Violet Tourmaline, Alexandrite, Clear Quartz Crystal, Danburite

Clears and opens crown chakra obstructions and blockages, repairs karmic damage to the crown; facilitates understanding and releasing negative karmic patterns, assists in karmic release, enhances past life regression work; promotes working with the Lords of karma and accessing one's karmic records (Akashic Records) for releasing karmic patterns, promotes karmic and spiritual level core soul healing; increases psychic abilities, helps communication with spirit guides, assists in spiritual evolution and attaining enlightenment, aids all spirituality

JACOBENIA
(Jacobenia sp.)
(Heart) Pink

> **Add Gemstones:** Mangano Calcite, Pink Calcite, Pink tourmaline, Pink Andean Opal, Pink Coral, Kunzite, Pink Sapphire, Peach Moonstone, Herkimer Diamond, Danburite

> Promotes a joyful heart, creates heart's ease, fosters having a peaceful heart and mind; promotes emotional heart healing of all kinds, releases heart scars gently, makes the heart bloom with joy; increases one's ability to feel and express love and trust, helps in validating and feeling emotion in oneself and others; helps in moving through the grief process, increases understanding and acceptance, assists in going on with one's life

JAPANESE TOAD LILY
(Tricyrtis tojen)
(Heart) Pink

> **Add Gemstones:** Lepidolite, Lepidolite with Mica, Pink Tourmaline, Raspberry Garnet, Pink Fluorite, Pink Smithsonite, Pink Chinese Opal, Herkimer Diamond, Danburite

> Promotes freedom of heart and free spirits, supports living free of restrictions and unnecessary bounds, helps in being true to oneself and one's life path; helps in standing up to mediocrity and conformity; promotes following one's heart and one's soul knowing, aids in serving oneself and the planet; fosters a commitment to truth and purity, aids in knowing and following one's inner truth

JASMINE, Carolina
(Gelsemium sempervirens)

(Solar Plexus) Yellow

> **Add Gemstones:** Yellow Kyanite, Amber, Amber Calcite, Yellow Zincite, Dravite, Septarian, Lemon Yellow Calcite, Clear Quartz Crystal, Danburite
>
> Increases energy, will and strength; promotes a zest for living, encourages a new appreciation of life everyday; increases and encourages the will to live, reduces lethargy and apathy; cleanses, clears and heals the kundalini chakras and kundalini line; provides emotional support for those with debilitating dis-eases; increases the eagerness and joy in one's life. Also called Yellow Jasmine or Gelsemium.

JASMINE, Confederate
(Trachelospermum jasminoides)

(Hara) White

> **Add Gemstones:** Peach Aventurine, Orange Calcite, Mexican Opal, Jelly Opal, Peach Moonstone, White Moonstone, White Opal, Carnelian, Orange Sunstone, Herkimer Diamond, Danburite
>
> Completes and fulfills the union of body and soul between love partners, enhances love's physical and spiritual consummation, joins twin souls and twin flames; aids harmony and total peace together, promotes marriage for life and beyond; provides karmic healing between lovers and soul mates, enhances and aids lovers' mutual commitment together; celebrates the beloved

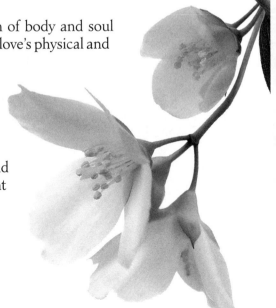

JERUSALEM THORN TREE
(Parkinsonia aculeata)

(Solar Plexus) Yellow

> **Add Gemstones:** Golden Beryl, Golden Topaz, Sunstone, Lemon Yellow Calcite, Green Calcite, Peridot, Tiger Eye, Yellow Jade, Green Jade, Clear Quartz Crystal, Danburite
>
> Stimulates the powers and abilities of the mind; promotes intellect, intuition, learning and studying, creativity, psychic awareness and psychic abilities; encourages openness to new ideas, promotes mental growth and expansion; cleanses, heals and repairs the mental body and Mind Grid (higher level mental body); stimulates astral travel and healing dreams; aids and increases mental and psychic receptivity and self-awareness. Also called Jelly Bean Tree.

KAPOK TREE
(Bomliax ceilia)

(Root) Red

> **Add Gemstones:** Ruby, Star Ruby, Garnet, Spinel, Elestial Smoky Quartz, Black Velvet Tourmaline, Rainbow Obsidian, Black Kyanite, Herkimer Diamond, Danburite
>
> Heals all aspects of women's sexuality, helps in healing past sexual abuse; stimulates the life force, restores love of living, strengthens the will to live, assists survival issues; promotes kundalini opening, grounds and balances rising kundalini energy, stabilizes energy flows; clears stagnant energy, clears situations of being stuck, promotes needed transformation in one's life

KING'S MANTLE
(Thunbergia erecta)

(Crown) Purple and Gold

> **Add Gemstones:** Rutile Amethyst, Ametrine, Rutile Citrine, Purple Fluorite, Sugilite, Charoite, Violet Tourmaline, Gold Fluorite, Alexandrite, Clear Quartz Crystal, Danburite
>
> Balances spiritual opening with daily living, balances the psychic realm with the conscious earth plane mind; calms new psychics and those experiencing an acceleration of psychic energies, aids those who fear their psychic knowledge and what they perceive; stabilizes new channelers, controls rising kundalini energies

LANTANA
(Lantana camara)

(Crown) Lavender and White

> **Add Gemstones:** Charoite, Amethyst, Amethyst Quartz, Purple Fluorite, Sugilite, Rainbow Moonstone, Lepidolite, Phenacite, Herkimer Diamond, Danburite
>
> Provides energy stabilization during transformative processes; helps in past life regression and understanding the lessons of past lives, promotes working with the Lords of Karma; helps in consciously connecting one's emotions to their karmic sources, opens and releases negative karmic emotional patterns; promotes understanding the karmic plan for one's life, soothes and calms

LANTANA
(Lantana camara)

(Belly and Solar Plexus) Orange and Gold

> **Add Gemstones:** Amber, Vanadanite, Honey Calcite, Natural Citrine, Carnelian, Red Jasper, Jelly Opal, Mexican Opal, Clear Quartz Crystal, Danburite
>
> Provides energetic stability, helps in connecting emotions to their sources, helps in understanding "what happened"; aids in releasing old and unprocessed this-life traumas, releases and removes the trauma pictures stored in the belly chakra; may promote an emotional release (crying, anger, talking about the trauma, laughing); eases the process of release, reduces anxiety, an emotional rescue essence

LANTANA
(Lantana camara)

(Heart and Solar Plexus) Pink and Yellow

> **Add Gemstones:** Rhodochrosite, Amber, Pink Kunzite, Lepidolite with Mica, Pink Fluorite, Yellow Fluorite, Yellow Opal, Honey Calcite, Citrine, Clear Quartz Crystal, Danburite

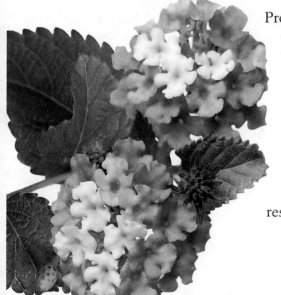

> Promotes the stability of all energy systems; aids accessing and processing one's emotions, can cause a needed emotional release and clearing; helps to process and release present-life traumas especially those that are old and have never been healed; helps in relieving and releasing stress, protects and insulates; an emotional rescue essence

LARKSPUR
(Delphinium elatum Chocolate)
(Grounding) Brown

> **Add Gemstones:** Brown Jasper, Boulder Opal, Staurolite, Ammonite Fossil, Brown Agate, Petrified Wood, Crazy Lace Jasper, Smoky Quartz, Clear Quartz Crystal, Danburite
>
> For planting one's feet deeply into Mother Earth, promotes coming fully into the physical, being rooted and grounded, develops one's connections to the planet; develops the hara line grounding system, connects one's grounding cord and grounding system firmly and properly into the core of the Earth; provides security and stability, promotes practicality and responsibility; makes it safe to do out of body work because you are fully connected, brings astral travelers back into their bodies and back to Earth, provides grounding and centering; protects

LARKSPUR
(Delphinium depauperatum ranunculaceae)
(Third Eye) Dark blue

> **Add Gemstones:** Azurite, Azurite-Chrysocolla, Azurite-Malachite, Blue Dumortierite, Lapis Lazuli, Blue Sapphire, Sodalite, Iolite, Blue Coral, Clear Quartz Crystal, Danburite
>
> For overcoming fickleness in oneself, promotes taking life more seriously, encourages being responsible and reliable; aids the inability to concentrate, increases mental focus, increases the desire and ability to study, increases focus on spirituality and spiritual studies, offers the gift of psychic opening for those who earn it. Larkspur is also called Delphinium; it symbolizes levity and lightness in the Victorian flower language.

LARKSPUR
(Consolida ambigua)
(Heart) Pink

> **Add Gemstones:** Rose Quartz, Pink Kunzite, Purple Kunzite, Mangano Calcite, Pink Calcite, Morganite, Pink Tourmaline, Clear Quartz Crystal, Danburite
>
> Centers spiritual opening in the heart chakra; provides psychic ability and information especially for healers and hospice workers and those who work with babies and animals; promotes self-healing, increases one's abilities as a healer and self-heale; encourages emotional maturity without the loss of joy, assists all emotional healing; helps those afraid of aging or dying

LAVENDER
(Lavendula officinalis)
(Crown) Purple

> **Add Gemstones:** Spirit Quartz, Violet Tourmaline, Sugilite, Purple Kunzite, Lepidolite, Amethyst, Amethyst with Hematite, Herkimer Diamond, Danburite
>
> Facilitates one's contact and work with the Lords of Karma and Akashic Records (the soul's past life records); promotes karmic release and healing of karmic damage, heals trauma and negativity from past lives, heals negative karmic patterns and suffering, releases karmic attachments and blockages to the crown; aids and stabilizes during Essential Energy Balancing processes and all ascension work; promotes all spirituality, increases one's spiritual evolution while soothing the way, promotes enlightenment (ascension) in this lifetime

LIGNUM VITAE TREE
(Guaiacum officinale)
(Thymus) Blue

> **Add Gemstones:** Blue Opal, Blue Andean Opal, Lapis Lazuli, Blue Dumortierite, Eilat Stone, Turquoise, Azurite-Chrysocolla, Azurite, Herkimer Diamond, Danburite
>
> Promotes self-healing and all healing; regenerates, heals and repairs the energy bodies especially the mental body, stabilizes the immune system at the emotional body level; promotes all magickal workings—Merlin's staff was said to be made of this tree, increases consciousness and mental control, enhances creativity; also helps and heals past abuse, reduces stress, cools and soothes, lessens grief, calms restlessness, increases concentration, aids insomnia

LILAC
(Syringa vulgaris)
(Crown) Purple

> **Add Gemstones:** Alexandrite, Amethyst, Amethyst Quartz, Violet Tourmaline, Lepidoite with Mica, Charoite, Purple Fluorite, Spirit Quartz, Clear Quartz Crystal, Danburite
>
> Awakens love—spiritual love, idealized love, love of Goddess or God, soulful love; promotes an appreciation of the soul and of the spiritual life, promotes acceptance of spiritual growth, encourages seeing the sacred in the everyday; fosters openness to new people, situations and things; aids life stage transitions; good essence for children becoming adolescents and adolescents reaching adulthood; encourages flexibility, acceptance of change, mental relaxation, reduces stress and provides peaceful sleep

LILAC
(Syringa vulgaris)
(Crown) White

> **Add Gemstones:** Phenacite, Selenite, White Opal, Fire Opal, White Moonstone, Rainbow Moonstone, Stilbite, Snow Quartz, White Apophyllite, Clear Quartz Crystal, Danburite
>
> Assists the ending of love affairs, provides gentle movement between life stages and love relationships; helps to sustain young love, first love, heals love's ending for all ages but especially the end of a first affair; turns infatuation into real love when appropriate, sustains marriage or long term relationships; supports and enhances feminine energy and feminine transformations; assists life's transitions of all kinds. White Lilac is a traditional symbol for innocence.

LILY, Easter
(Lilium sp.)
(Crown) White

> **Add Gemstones:** Golden Topaz, Champagne Topaz, Citrine, Amber, Lemon Yellow Calcite, Yellow Sapphire, Golden Beryl, Selenite, Phenacite, Clear Quartz Crystal, Danburite
>
> Eases and protects through life changes and transitions, supports all the rites of passage but especially birth and death; offers peaceful dying at one's proper time to die, heals despair and fear, promotes letting go, promotes trust in Goddess and all of life's (and death's) processes, encourages knowledge of past lives and that we have been here before; fills the chakras and bodies with Light, promotes enlightenment, protects those entering and leaving incarnation; helps to stabilize newborns

LILY, Lollipop
(Lilium sp.)
(Heart) Pink and White

> **Add Gemstones:** Mangano Calcite, Pink Sapphire, Gem Rose Quartz, Pink Fluorite, Kunzite, Morganite, White Moonstone, Pfeach Moonstone, Herkimer Diamond, Danburite
>
> Awakens the heart to the joys of living, soothes and heals the heart, reveals joy where there seems to be none; offers hope, calm and inner peace, promotes optimism and the will to continue; aids grief, depression, heartache, loneliness, and sadness

LILY, Spider
— *See SPIDER LILY*

LILY, Stargazer
(Lilium speciosum rubrum)
(Transpersonal Point) Purple and White

> **Add Gemstones:** Charoite, Sugilite, Moldavite, Canadian Amethyst, Alexandrite, Purple Sapphire, Violet Tourmaline, Phenacite, Herkimer Diamond, Danburite
>
> Assists and encourages reaching for the stars; promotes contact with Star Goddesses and guides, intergalactic healers, other-planetary healers; promotes psychic contact and reception of information from other planets and dimensions; supports contact and learning from one's oversoul; helps and protects those who astral travel or have astral relationships; good essence for astrologers and astronomers, helps channelers

LILY, Tiger
— *See TIGER LILY*

LILY, White Angel
(Lilium sp.)

(Transpersonal Point) White

> **Add Gemstones:** Seraphanite, Angelite, Angel Wing Selenite, Phenacite, Rainbow Moonstone, White or Fire Opal, Clear Beryl, White Topaz, Diamond, Herkimer Diamond, Danburite

> Promotes all contact with the angelic realm and their guidance and protection; aids in becoming an angel in oneself, promotes connecting and merging with one's angelic levels— Higher Self, Essence Self, Goddess Self; heals and connects the DNA, facilitates core soul healing at spiritual body and causal body levels (higher soul levels), repairs the silver cord that connects spirit and body and keeps one alive; heals and repairs the heart complex (heart on all levels) and heart complex connections; promotes ascension

LILY OF THE NILE
(Agapantha)

(Third Eye) Blue

> **Add Gemstones:** Blue Tourmaline, Lapis Lazuli, Azurite, Blue Aventurine, Blue Sapphire, Celestite, Angelite, Phenacite, Clear Quartz Crystal, Danburite

> Stimulates the third eye especially for psychic healers; increases the ability to see psychically and to interpret and use what is seen, helps one to become a competent psychic healer; brings in psychic information strongly, increases and stimulates all psychic abilities, promotes rapid psychic development that may be too fast to be comfortable; aids the transitions and changes of Reiki II; promotes clairvoyance and crystal gazing, aids meditation, past life regression, all forms of psychic healing

LILY OF THE VALLEY
(Convallaria majalis)

(All Aura) White

> **Add Gemstones:** Violet Tourmaline, Iolite, Celestite, Watermelon Tourmaline, Rose Quartz, Amber, Citrine, Pecos Quartz, Garnet, Herkimer Diamond, Danburite
>
> Provides energy protection for infants, children, teenagers, and pets; protects the innocence and security of those new to the world; promotes feeling safe, loved, secure and wanted; good for children in daycare, kindergarten or school, good for pets while boarding; helps children and pets on trips to strange places or to the doctor or vet; prevents nightmares and other fear situations. Symbolizes return of happiness in the Victorian flower language.

LISIANTHUS
(Eustoma grandiflorum)

(Crown) Purple

> **Add Gemstones:** Spirit Quartz, Purple Druzy Quartz, Amethyst, Rutile Amethyst, Canadian Amethyst, Sugilite, Lepidolite, Purple Fluorite, Clear Quartz Crystal, Danburite
>
> Calms and soothes, promotes a quiet mind, reduces mental chatter, aids the inability to still the mind and quiet the body; promotes trust in the Goddess and spirituality especially in times of adversity or trauma, heals this-life and past-life emotional traumas; provides peace, comfort, hope and spiritual healing, eases fear; reduces insomnia, nightmares and restless sleep; use as an emotional rescue in times of stress or pain

LOBELIA
(Lobelia chinensis)
(Third Eye) Blue

> **Add Gemstones:** Blue Sapphire, Azurite, Blue Kyanite, Lapis Lazuli, Azurite-Chrysocolla, Celestite, Blue Kunzite, Holly Blue Agate, Blue Labradorite, Herkimer Diamond, Danburite

> Accelerates psychic opening and development—sometimes roughly, shatters emotional and mental barriers to growth and achievement on all levels, may be rough but is always of the Light; aids in gaining the assistance of spirit guides, angels, Lords of Karma and Goddess in one's process of growth and change; pushes forward those who are lazy or too timid to make spiritual progress, ends procrastination and avoidance; aids in rebirthing, sometimes causes spontaneous rebirth; initiates transformations on all levels, all healing

LOOSESTRIFE
(Lythrum salicaria)
(Third Eye) Blue

> **Add Gemstones:** Azurite, Lapis Lazuli, Blue Aventurine, Blue Sapphire, Iolite, Sodalite, Blue Labradorite, Blue Pietersite, Shattuckite, Herkimer Diamond, Danburite

> Opens the third eye and initiates psychic opening; shows what one's psychic skills and abilities are, increases psychic potential, increases psychic images and information; heals the third eye chakra and crown, heals the connections between the third eye and crown, opens the throat chakra; makes psychic perception possible, promotes clairvoyance and channeling, promotes visualization ability, increases all psychic abilities; provides connection with spirit guides, angels, Lords of Karma, alien healers, Goddess and the Light; puts one on a path of learning and spirituality

LOOSESTRIFE
(Lythrum salicaria)
(Causal Body) Red-Violet

> **Add Gemstones:** Pink Tourmaline, Violet Tourmaline, Kyanite with Rubellite, Blue Kyanite, Amethyst, Sugilite, Lepidolite, Lepidolite with Mica, Herkimer Diamond, Danburite
>
> Develops, heals, rewires and reprograms the causal body chakra; evolves one to ascension and enlightenment levels, enables and opens advanced psychic abilities of information reception; provides connection to high level Light Be-ings for instruction and teaching, brings advanced spiritual information through to be used for good; promotes connection with Goddess, Lords of Karma, high level alien helpers and healers, and other Light Be-ings; strengthens psychic reception and channeling, aids automatic writing, inspires psychic intuition of advanced healing information

LOOSESTRIFE
(Lysimachia punctata)
(Hara) Golden Yellow

> **Add Gemstones:** Amber, Tiger Eye, Golden Beryl, Natural Citrine, Yellow Kyanite, Champagne Topaz, Dravite (Golden Tourmaline), Yellow Sapphire, Sunstone, Herkimer Diamond, Danburite
>
> Centers life force energy (ch'i) in the hara chakra, fills the entire hara line with Light and healing; removes obstructions and blockages, releases negative cords and hooks from all the chakras of the hara line, cleanses and purifies; repairs and reprograms the mental body and mind grid (higher level of the mental body) and their chakras; centers the incarnation on one's karmic life purpose, brings energy to one's life purpose, assists in discovering one's true life path, facilitates every aspect of its expression; provides guidance and help in manifesting and fulfilling one's life purpose, promotes fulfillment and joy

MAGNOLIA
(Magnolia grandiflora)
(Crown) White

>**Add Gemstones:** Diamond, Selenite, White Phantom Calcite, Clear Calcite, White Moonstone, White Druzy Quartz, Clear Beryl, White Topaz, Herkimer Diamond, Danburite
>
>Promotes spiritual and psychic opening, increases psychic growth, fosters psychic awakening; assists in learning all psychic and spirituality skills and in learning how to apply and use them; promotes connection with spirit guides, nonphysical teachers and Goddess, enhances psychic communication and learning; aid to experiencing awareness levels beyond the physical, promotes a new way of thinking and Be-ing, promotes self-awareness, promotes self-confidence and self-assurance

MANDEVILLA
(Mandevilla splendens)
(Heart) Pink

>**Add Gemstones:** Mangano Calcite, Gem Rose Quartz, Kunzite, Pink Tourmaline, Pink Andean Opal, Pink Chinese Opal, Rhodonite, Pink Sapphire, Herkimer Diamond, Danburite
>
>For heart healing on all levels, eases heartache and heartbreak, promotes emotional healing and release, intiates gentle clearing and release of heart scars; heals past and current this-life abuse, clears and heals past-life abuse and abuse patterns, releases and heals karmic patterns of heartbreak and betrayal; promotes positive self worth and joy in living, eases grief, regret and self-blame

MARIGOLD
(Calendula officinalis)
(Belly) Yellow Orange

> **Add Gemstones:** Jelly Opal, Fire Opal, Orange Calcite, Honey Calcite, Lemon Yellow Calcite, Carnelian, Carnelian Agate, Mookite, Clear Quartz Crystal, Danburite
>
> Soothes the emotions and the mind, calms, promotes acceptance, encourages inner peace; reduces sexual lust, good for balancing teens with newly awakening sexual needs, promotes sexual responsibility, increases the ability to wait; can stimulate psychic dreams and psychic visions of magickal creatures (like unicorns and griffins). Also called Calendula, symbolizes grief and despair in the language of flowers.

MONKS' ASTER
(Aster sp.)
(Throat) Blue

> **Add Gemstones:** Blue Tourmaline, Blue Lace Agate, Turquoise, Blue Aventurine, Angelite, Celestite, Lapis Lazuli, Sodalite, Clear Quartz Crystal, Herkimer Diamond
>
> Clears obstructions and blockages in the throat, third eye and thymus chakras; releases and heals negative karma and karmic obstructions from this life and past incarnations, releases harmful karmic patterns; aids in understanding and expressing one's karmic and personal truths; enhances the ability and creativity to express and manifest one's life purpose, promotes certainty on one's life path; stimulates gentle psychic opening, increases inner knowing, enhances calm inner peace

MOONFLOWER
(Ipomea sp.)

(Hara) White

> **Add Gemstones:** Peach Moonstone, Mexican Opal, Jelly Opal, Peach Calcite, Peach Aventurine, Golden Lace Jasper, Amber, Clear Quartz Crystal, Danburite
>
> Brings psychic information and awareness into consciousness and earth plane clarity, helps in understanding and interpreting psychic information and how to use it practically; encourages psychic opening and development, improves meditation and all psychic study; clears and opens the hara line chakras; increases contact with spirit guides, angels, Goddess and the Light; helps in finding and achieving one's life purpose and life path, stabilizes one's life path

MORNING GLORY
(Ipomea learu)

(Third Eye) Blue

> **Add Gemstones:** Blue Aventurine, Holly Blue Agate, Aqua Aura Crystal, Celestite, Larimar, Lapis Lazuli, Iolite, Blue Opal, Clear Quartz Crystal, Danburite
>
> Initiates travel to far places, other dimensions and planets; promotes astral travel, meditation, guided meditation, psychic journeys; expands and heals the mind and mental body, cleanses, repairs, connects; aids linking into the collective consciousness of the planet as an information library; provides contact with Light Be-ings, positive alien healers and teachers, Goddess, nature devas; encourages mental telepathy and communication with dolphins, animals, people; promotes psychic awareness of other realms

MULLEIN
(Verbascum thapsus)
(Solar Plexus) Yellow

> **Add Gemstones:** Citrine, Lemon Yellow Calcite, Yellow Fluorite, Yellow Jade, Yellow Opal, Yellow Sapphire, Septarian, Tiger Eye, Clear Quartz Crystal, Danburite
>
> Cleanses and purifies the solar plexus chakra and entire kundalini line, clears and washes the aura and auric field, fills the chakras and channels with Light; fills the aura with Light and healing, expands the auric envelope, clears dark areas and cloudy patches in the aura; increases assimilation of Light energy, increases reception of psychic information; expands the mind, promotes clear thinking and new ideas, relaxes and aids concentration

MULLEIN, Caribbean Crush
(Verbascum Caribbean Crush)
(Heart, Solar Plexus, Belly) Pink, Yellow, Peach

> **Add Gemstones:** Use one of each color--Rose Quartz, Kunzite, Pink Calcite; Lemon Yellow Calcite, Citrine, Yellow Jade; Peach Moonstone, Honey Calcite, Champagne Topaz; Herkimer Diamond, Danburite
>
> Clears the connections and interactions between the heart, solar plexus and belly chakras; heals and balances the chakras and the kundalini line, heals the rotation and spin of the chakras; fills the aura and auric field with Light and expands the auric envelope, heals the emotional body; unifies the emotions (heart), mind (solar plexus) and physical levels (belly), promotes an open heart, clear mind, and stable body; increases joy and well-being, and an optimistic outlook

NAKED LADY
(Lycoris squamigera)
(Heart Complex) Pink

> **Add Gemstones:** Lepidolite, Pink Fluorite, Pink Kunzite, Purple Kunzite, Rose Quartz, Pink Sapphire, Selenite, Fire Opal, Herkimer Diamond, Danburite
>
> Primarily a women's essence; opens and activates the heart complex (heart on all levels) chakras and channels, repairs damage to the silver cord that connects the physical body to life; promotes love on all levels—universal love, unconditional love, compassionate love, sexual love, nurturing love; encourages the giving and receiving of love of all kinds; promotes self-love, positive self-image, positive body image; assists in forgiving oneself and others; supports spiritual growth on all levels and of all types, promotes becoming a bodhisattva on Earth and attaining enlightenment (or ascension) in this lifetime; heals grief. Also called Resurrection Lily, Naked Nun, Rain Lily or Magic Lily.

NARCISSUS, February Gold
(Narsissus sp.)
(Solar Plexus) Yellow

> **Add Gemstones:** Yellow Opal, Yellow Fluorite, Rutile Citrine, Yellow Calcite, Golden Labradorite, Golden Beryl, Yellow Jade, Moonstone, Clear Quartz Crystal, Danburite
>
> For healthy self-confidence and positive self-image, balances the ego, offers clarity; supports positive boundaries, aids in being appropriately open to others, increases one's caring and courtesy toward others and oneself, aids in being considerate and cooperative toward others; promotes living in harmony with oneself and one's world

NARCISSUS, Golden Ducat
(Narcissus sp.)
(Solar Plexus) Yellow

Add Gemstones: Peridot, Green Kunzite, Green Calcite, Green Amber, Green Tourmaline, Emerald, Green Siberian Quartz, Herkimer Diamond, Danburite

Promotes finding one's place in the physical world, encourages self-confidence in earth plane activities of all kinds, promotes working cooperatively with others; focuses on the Zen of daily living and spiritual consciousness in daily life, makes daily life into a spiritual exercise, supports spiritual evolution through everyday physical action; balances the will and ego, encourages physical prosperity and spiritual abundance

NARCISSUS, Paperwhite
(Narcissus tazetta)
(Thymus) White

Add Gemstones: Turquoise, Celestite, Blue Andean Opal, Blue Opal, Larimar, Blue Tourmaline, Kyanite, Aquamarine, Amazonite, Herkimer Diamond, Danburite

Promotes a harmony of inner and outer Be-ing, balances and harmonizes daily living with living a spiritual life; aids living as a conscious spiritual Be-ing in the earth plane world; promotes clearing the emotions and emotional attachments, releasing emotional karma; accelerates spiritual evolution and growth, supports those on the path to enlightenment or ascension; increases one's awareness of beauty and perfection in one's life, increases happiness and joy; heals the higher levels of the heart and heart complex. In the flower language and in Roman mythology, Narcissus symbolizes egotism; as an essence it changes egotism to humility.

NASTURTIUM
(Tropaeolum majus)

(Vision) Cream

Add Gemstones: Seraphanite, Sugilite, Yellow Fluorite, Phantom Quartz, Clear Fluorite, Grey Moonstone, White Moonstone, Labradorite, Phenacite, Herkimer Diamond, Danburite

Balances the left and right hemispheres of the brain, balances the mental with the spiritual, focuses the mind for learning and spiritual work, filters psychic static; heals and balances the mental body, aligns and opens the mental body chakras; promotes mental effort, reduces mind chatter; aids psychic vision and visions, aids channeling, aids crystal gazing and scrying, promotes all psychic work

NIGHTBLOOMING CEREUS
(Cereus peruvianus)

(Third Eye) White

Add Gemstones: Moonstone, Blue Opal, Blue Chalcedony, Lapis Lazuli, Azurite, Selenite, Phenacite, White Coral, Girasol Quartz, Clear Quartz Crystal, Danburite

For the Moon, Moon Goddesses and Moon Rituals, aids in Drawing Down the Moon in ritual, focuses lunar cycles and lunar energies; promotes connection with individual Moon Goddesses (Hathor, Isis, Selene, The Lady); also promotes connecting with the stars, star constellations, star rituals, and Star Goddesses; amplifies all psychic work, supports meditation; harmonizes women's bodies to the cycles of the moon and stars, accesses moon wisdom and women's mysteries, accesses the mysteries of the night and the stars, aphrodisiac

ORANGE BLOSSOM
(Citrus sinensis)
(Heart) White

Add Gemstones: Pink Sapphire, Pink Druzy Quartz, Rose Quartz, Pink Kunzite, Pink Tourmaline, Cobaltite, Diamond, Herkimer Diamond, Clear Quartz Crystal, Danburite

Heals heart scars and brings about emotional release—more gently than is usual, provides all heart healing; promotes enlightened relationships, twin soul relationships, long term relationships and marriage; increases trust and positive self-esteem, reduces codependency, aids the ability to follow your heart with regard to relationships and more; provides clarity and calming, eases depression from lost love, reduces anxiety. Traditional definition is the marriage wreath and chastity, purity and fidelity.

ORCHID, Dancing Lady
(Oncidium sp.)
(Hara) Yellow and Red

Add Gemstones: Rhodochrosite, Gem Rhodochrosite, Red Jasper, Yellow Jasper, Mookite, Amber, Moroccan Red Quartz, Vanadinite, Clear Quartz Crystal, Danburite

Promotes light feet and a light heart, helps in seeing life as a joyful dance, provides the ability to take joy in life and appreciate life's lighter side; aids those who work too hard and forget how to play, reduces stress, promotes slowing down and taking time off to have fun, aids workaholics and those too serious to laugh; promotes laughter, joy, playfulness and fun

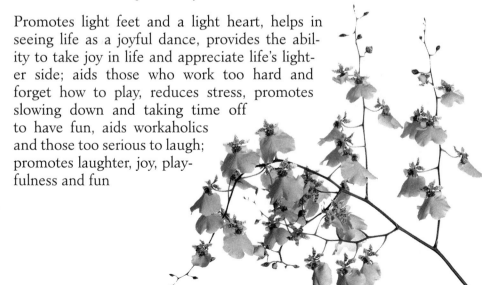

ORCHID, MOTH
(Phalaenopsis sp.)
(Heart) Pink

> **Add Gemstones:** Pink Andean Opal, Pink Chinese Opal, Rose Quartz, Pink Sapphire, Ruby, Rhodonite, Raspberry Garnet, Pink Calcite, Herkimer Diamond, Danburite
>
> Aids in making contact and learning to work with members of the fairy realm, plant and garden devas, gemstone devas; promotes communication from and through the heart, increases trust and openness in interactions with other-dimensional nature Be-ings; creates a protected state of interaction and sharing, assists cooperation and co-creation, promotes innocence; good essence for those who work as Earth healers or planetary caretakers

OXALIS
(Oxalis valicola)
(Heart) Pink

> **Add Gemstones:** Lepidolite, Mangano Calcite, Pink Kunzite, Purple Kunzite, Pink Jade, Rose Quartz, Pink Smithsonite, Herkimer Diamond, Danburite
>
> Clears, heals and opens the heart; repairs damage to the heart chakra and heart complex of chakras, repairs this-life and past life damage to the emotional and astral (higher emotional) bodies; increases one's ability to make secure decisions and choices, soothes and calms, promotes inner peace; helps those with anxiety, insomnia, worry, insecurity, anger. Also called Wood Sorrel or Wild Oxalis.

OXALIS
(Oxalis oregona)
(All Chakras) White

> **Add Gemstones:** Phenacite, Snow Quartz, White Opal, Fire Opal, White Marble, Rainbow Moonstone, White Moonstone, Selenite, Clear Quartz Crystal, Danburite
>
> Use with all white or clear gemstones as an all-system cleanser, purifier and healer; balances, aligns, clears, repairs, opens all the chakras of the kundalini and hara lines; helps to heal core soul damage, heals aura tears, holes and other damage from this life and past lifetimes; heals damage received while coming into body to incarnate or while leaving the body at death; soothes, calms, brings inner peace, reduces anxiety and worry, promotes clarity in one's life and choices, promotes connection to the Goddess and the Light. Also called Wood Sorrel or Wild Oxalis.

OXALIS
(Oxalis albicans)
(Solar Plexus) Yellow

> **Add Gemstones:** Yellow Jade, Yellow Fluorite, Yellow Jasper, Yellow Kyanite, Natural Citrine, Golden Amber, Golden Beryl, Clear Beryl, Phenacite, Danburite
>
> Cleanses, clears, heals; aligns and opens the mental body and mind grid (higher mental levels) and all mental level chakras, repairs this-life and past life damage to the mental body levels; increases mental assimilation of all kinds (ideas, learning ability, energy reception, psychic information); provides mental soothing and calms the mind to stimulate inner peace, helps in "making up your mind", helps to promote clear and lucid choices and responsible decisions; reduces anxiety, worry, mental chatter, vacillation, anger, fear. Also called Wood Sorrel or Wild Oxalis.

PANDORA VINE
(Podranea ricasoliana)

(Heart) Lavender

> **Add Gemstones:** Pink Fluorite, Lepidolite, Lepidolite with Mica, Pink Jade, Pink Calcite, Kunzite, Mangano Calcite, Amethyst, Herkimer Diamond, Danburite
>
> Offers hope for every aspect of one's life, encourages trust in the Light and the Goddess, promotes trust in life and in love; repairs and regenerates the emotional body and astral body (higher level emotional) auras; provides emotional healing, heals the inner child, encourages healing between mother and child; encourages emotional stability, promotes peace of mind and heart, balances, calms; relieves despair, loneliness, hopelessness and loss

PANDORA VINE
(Pandora ricasoliana)

(Perineum) Red

> **Add Gemstones:** Red Zincite, Amethyst with Hematite, Ruby, Star Ruby, Red Phantom Calcite, White Calcite, Phenacite, Clear Quartz Crystal, Danburite
>
> Balances the spiritual with the Earthly, aids in being a psychic in the material world, promotes grounded earth plane functioning with open psychic abilities; stimulates psychic opening and development, increases psychic abilities and helps in learning to use them; helps in validating one's psychic abilities and perceptions, reduces fear of psychic impressions in new psychics; aids returning to Earth after psychic work, prevents spaciness, balances kundalini rising

PANSY, Delta Pure Red
(viola x wittrockiana)
(Perineum) Red

Add Gemstones: Smoky Quartz, Elestial Quartz, Red Obsidian, Red Pietersite, Ruby, Star Ruby, Hematite, Amethyst with Hematite, Black Jade, Black Tourmaline, Clear Quartz Crystal, Danburite

Repairs karmic damage to the hara line and hara line chakras, repairs and heals the perineum chakra on the hara line; rewires the grounding system, connects the grounding cord to the core of the Earth; stabilizes the incarnation, grounds and centers; brings the life force into the bodies, balances the life force and reduces too much energy entering the physical, calms jittery people. Viola is another name for this flower; the Victorians used it to symbolize thought.

PANSY, Fame Primrose
(Viola x wittrockiana)
(Diaphragm) Yellow

Add Gemstones: Champagne Topaz, Yellow Topaz, Green Amber, Yellow Amber, Yellow Jade, Green Jade, Green Tourmaline, Dravite (Golden Tourmaline), Clear Quartz Crystal, Danburite

Cleanses the hara line and all the hara line chakras and channels, detoxifies and purifies; heals karmic emotional damage and releases past life traumas and suffering, makes one aware of past life situations that are toxic for this lifetime; promotes sudden change, initiates karmic flashbacks and revelations, promotes past life information and release. Also called Viola, symbolizes thought in the flower language.

PANSY, Wild
(Viola tricolor)

(Solar Plexus) Purple and Yellow

> **Add Gemstones:** Ametrine, Amethyst, Yellow Fluorite, Yellow Opal, Yellow Jade, Violet Jade, Violet Tourmaline, Dravite, Sugilite, Herkimer Diamond, Danburite
>
> Connects the mental and the spiritual, balances the magickal with the everyday; encourages spiritual awareness in people who are logic-oriented; spiritualizes one's daily life, brings spiritual awareness into everyday actions and thoughts; promotes spiritual awakening in people who are too mental; promotes balance in all things. Also called Johnny Jump Up; the Victorian flower language uses pansies to symbolize thought.

PAPERWHITE
—See NARCISSUS, Paperwhite

PASSION FLOWER
(Passiflora caereulea)

(Third Eye) Blue

> **Add Gemstones:** Holly Blue Agate, Tanzanite, Lapis Lazuli, Avalonite (Blue Druzy Chalcedony), Azurite, Azurite-Chrysocolla, Clear Quartz Crystal, Danburite
>
> Accesses and translates Pleiadian wisdom and Star wisdom for Earth understanding; provides contact with Light Be-ing helpers, healers and teachers from other planets and galaxies; increases communication, comprehension, channeling and automatic writing of other-planetary information; increases and opens psychic abilities of all kinds, promotes mediumship, meditation and dreamwork; fosters universal love, unconditional love, awareness of the oneness of all life

PASSION FLOWER
(Passiflora incarnata)

(Perineum) Red

> **Add Gemstones:** Red Siberian Quartz, Garnet, Ruby, Star Ruby, Spinel, Black Tourmaline, Jet, Obsidian, Red Obsidian, Herkimer Diamond, Danburite
>
> Stimulates the life force and will to live, heals the life force in individuals; connects and interconnects one's physical and spiritual lives, aids living one's spirituality on the earth plane, promotes making ones daily earth plane life intrinsically spiritual; helps in manifesting one's life purpose, promotes honoring the oneness of all life; offers spiritual protection, repels negativity, releases and ends attachments and negative entities; grounds after psychic work

PENSTEMON, Red Rocks
(Penstemon x mexicali)

(Perineum) Red

> **Add Gemstones:** Ruby, Star Ruby, Hematite, Amethyst with Hematite, Tourmaline Quartz, Moroccan Red Quartz, Red Jasper, Clear Quartz Crystal, Danburite
>
> Promotes excitement and anticipation, brings energy and zest back into one's life after trauma or debility; strengthens the life force, strengthens the will to live, increases one's joy in living; fills the kundalini and hara lines with life force (ch'i) energy, repairs and cleanses the perineum and root chakras, heals the physical level aura (etheric double); encourages the will to continue in worn out people, heals burnout, heals those who wonder if life is worth living, heals the sad and empty. Also called Bearded Tongue.

PENSTEMON, Shadow Mountain
(Penstemon x mexicali)

(Crown) Violet and Red

Add Gemstones: Sugilite, Violet Tourmaline, Holly Blue Agate, Amethyst, Amethyst with Hematite, Amethyst Quartz, Spirit Quartz, Purple Druzy Quartz, Herkimer Diamond, Danburite

Connects the physical and spiritual with the focus on bringing the spiritual into physical form; promotes interest in spirituality, encourages spiritual awakening; pushes those who resist their spiritual natures into accepting and recognizing who they are, stops resistance and refusal; works to make one's life spiritual no matter what one does on the physical, makes everyday living into a spiritual exercise, makes people aware that they are more than physical; soothes the deep transformations that it causes. Also called Bearded Tongue.

PENTAS
(Pentas lanceolata)

(Causal Body) Pink

Add Gemstones: Dolomite, Petalite, Pink Andean Opal, Rose Quartz, Pink Sapphire, Pink Calcite, Mangano Calcite, Pink Coral, Herkimer Diamond, Danburite

Promotes receiving wisdom from the Star Goddess, accesses contact with star guides, helps in receiving and understanding information and wisdom from the galaxy and stars; a very good energy for Wiccan rituals, aids in Drawing down the Stars in ritual; increases the power of psychic work, aids channeling information from very far away, increases the range of astral travel, promotes advanced spirituality practices

PENTAS
(Pentas lanceolata)
(Causal Body) Red-Violet

> **Add Gemstones:** Spirit Quartz, Kunzite, Cobaltite, Gem Rose Quartz, Pink Sapphire, Violet Tourmaline, Raspberry Garnet, Herkimer Diamond, Danburite
>
> Assists in the development and opening of the causal body chakra on the hara line; promotes contact and reception of information from Goddess, Lords of Karma, angels, spirit guides and other-planetary Light energies; connects one to the Star Goddesses and star guides, aids in receiving star wisdom and information from the stars; aids in reception and channeling of information from high level galactic Be-ings; aids in consciousness of universal truths, promotes awareness of Earth's place in the universe

PEONY
(Paeonia lactiflora)
(Root) Dark Red

> **Add Gemstones:** Ruby, Star Ruby, Garnet, Amethyst with Hematite, Hematite, Moroccan Red Quartz, Cuprite, Clear Quartz Crystal, Danburite
>
> For grief recovery, assists in releasing and healing anger due to grief, aids moving through the stages of grief, promotes letting go; encourages the release and healing of blame and self-blame, fosters acceptance and forgiveness; sparks the will to live, promotes being grounded in the physical world, replaces anger with love

PEONY
(Paeonia lactiflora)

(Heart) Pink

> **Add Gemstones:** Pink Coral, Lazurine, Rose Quartz, Dolomite, Pink Kunzite, Morganite, Pink Calcite, Mangano Calcite, Pink Tourmaline, Clear Quartz Crystal, Danburite
>
> Heals grief especially for and about children; heals the shock of one's first great loss (of a person, pet, love affair, etc.), helps to heal an adult who has lost a child or a wanted pregnancy; aids moving through the process of grieving, aids in letting go, promotes understanding and acceptance; gives the ability to forgive and more forward; heals the loss of innocence, lifts depression, comforts and soothes, gentle energy healing

PEONY
(Paeonia lactiflora)

(Thymus) White

> **Add Gemstones:** Phenacite, White Moonstone, Rainbow Moonstone, Clear Topaz, Turquoise, Aquamarine, Larimar, Aqua Kyanite, Gem Silica, Herkimer Diamond, Danburite
>
> Heals grief by dissolving and releasing it, helps one to move through the stages of grief, prevents getting stuck or stopped in the grief process; heals guilt, blame, self-blame, resentment, and anger from grief; aids in letting go and letting Goddess, eases depression; promotes an awareness of the immortality of the soul, creates and fosters inner peace and acceptance

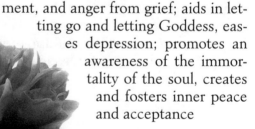

PETRA VINE
(Petra valubilis)

(Throat) Blue

> **Add Gemstones:** Azurite, Angelite, Celestite, Blue Chalcedony, Blue Pietersite, Amazonite, Lapis Lazuli, Blue Dumortierite, Herkimer Diamond, Danburite
>
> Brings calm and peace of mind, promote inner peace, inspires happiness, provides contentment with one's life; gives a feeling of wellness and the confidence that everything is good and right, offers a sense of well-being; increases connection with spirit guides and angels, increases connection with Goddess and the Light; heals and regenerates the Higher Self and the soul structure, promotes core soul healing; increases artistry and creativity, promotes speaking out and free expression; an essence for all-healing. Also called Bluebird Vine.

PINK MUHLY GRASS
(Muhlenbergia capillaris)

(Heart) Pink

> **Add Gemstones:** Pink Kunzite, Pink Smithsonite, Pink Sapphire, Pink Calcite, Pink Tourmaline, Watermelon Tourmaline, Rose Quartz, Herkimer Diamond, Danburite
>
> Inspires softness of heart, promotes easing a heart that has hardened from pain or disappointment; heals the heart chakra and heart complex (all levels of the heart), fills the kundalini line with love and peace; releases heart scars but may not do so gently; heals emotional pain as a sometimes-rough wake up call, promotes going forward in one's life without old scars and old emotional baggage; heals grudges and the need to hurt others

PINK POUI TREE
(Tabebuia pentaphylla)
(Heart) Pink

> **Add Gemstones:** Morganite, Lepidolite, Mangano Calcite, Pink Calcite, Pink Sapphire, Pink Tourmaline, Pink Andean Opal, Rose Quartz, Herkimer Diamond, Danburite
>
> For releasing and healing karmic pain patterns and their recurring this-life and past life damage; heals the heart chakra and heart complex (all the heart levels), heals the emotions and the emotional body; releases heart scars gently, offers an emotional wakeup call; eases heartache, heartbreak, emotional loss, despair, loneliness, grief; helps to return delight and happiness to living, promotes inner peace and joy

PLUMBAGO
(Plumbago capensis)
(Throat) Blue

> **Add Gemstones:** Angelite, Blue Lace Agate, Blue Kyanite, Blue Aventurine, Amazonite, Aquamarine, Turquoise, Celestite, Clear Quartz Crystal, Danburite
>
> Aids communication of all kinds; increases the ability to express personal emotional truths, releases anger from things unsaid, aids ability to express one's wants and needs, restores personal freedom by increasing positive assertiveness, good essence for those doing inner child work; strengthens psychic empathy, promotes connection and communication with spirit guides, angels, Lords of Karma and other Light guidance; increases creativity, releases artists' block, promotes calm and inner peace

POINCIANA, Dwarf
(Poinciana pulcherrima)
(Hara) Red and Yellow

> **Add Gemstones:** Red Pietersite, Red Tiger Eye, Spinel, Amber, Yellow Jade, Red Jasper, Yellow Sapphire, Ruby, Clear Quartz Crystal, Danburite
>
> For spiritual maturity; promotes coming into adulthood and adult responsibility, fosters sexual and emotional maturity; encourages manifesting one's life purpose on the earth plane, offers the energy to achieve and succeed in one's life purpose and in earth plane endeavors, limits procrastination and avoidance; promotes stability and taking charge, increases concentration and focus, encourages determination and serious intent

POINCIANA TREE
(Delonix regia)
(Perineum) Red and Gold

> **Add Gemstones:** Garnet, Ruby, Yellow Kyanite, Golden Beryl, Yellow Fluorite, Red Zincite, Yellow Zincite, Golden Labradorite, Herkimer Diamond, Danburite
>
> Supports and encourages the will to live, assists the desire to remain in the incarnation and stay on Earth; strengthens the life force, brings the soul firmly into the body; heals past life and this-life karma regarding giving up, suicide or leaving the lifetime too early; repairs and activates higher levels of the DNA; inspires determination to live and move forward despite all obstacles, promotes passion for living

POINCIANA TREE
(Peltophorum pterocarpum)
(Solar Plexus) Yellow

> **Add Gemstones:** Lemon Yellow Calcite, Natural Citrine, Yellow Siberian Quartz, Yellow Kyanite, Golden Topaz, Yellow Sapphire, Herkimer Diamond, Danburite
>
> For validating who you are, inspires recognizing personal truths, increases self-esteem and self-love; promotes self-awareness and self-confidence, protects vulnerable people; strengthens the will to live and the life force, initiates the will to continue and prevail; good essence for the transition from adolescence to adulthood, good for adults who were abused as children; assists those just staring out in life and becoming independent for the first time

POPPY, Carmen
(Papaver orientale)
(Root) Red

> **Add Gemstones:** Red Pietersite, Red Zincite, Ruby, Star Ruby, Garnet, Red Moroccan Quartz, Amethyst with Hematite, Clear Quartz Crystal, Danburite
>
> Stimulates the life force, brings increased life force energy through the kundalini line, can raise the kundalini (use Black Tourmaline to balance), pushes a strong force of energy through the kundalini chakras and channels; cleanses and clears the chakras, removes chakra obstructions, opens chakras that have previously been closed or blocked, increases chakra opening for already opened energy centers, flushes the aura with Light; puts one on their life path, ends resistance and procrastination, a cure for laziness and apathy. The Victorian flower language uses Red Poppy to denote fantastic extravagance!

POPPY, Manhattan
(Papaver orientale)
(Causal Body) Lavender

> **Add Gemstones:** Kyanite with Rubellite, Natural Star Sapphire, Lepidolite, Pink Druzy Quartz, Pink Tourmaline, Purple Kunzite, Sugilite, Violet Tourmaline, Herkimer Diamond, Danburite

> Develops and opens the causal body chakra on the hara line (emotional body), stimulates the spiritual evolution needed for the chakra to develop; intensifies one's path of spiritual opening and psychic development, increases psychic awareness, increases psychic and emotional empathy; initiates communication with the Light, puts one in contact and communication with positive discarnate entities of all kinds—Goddess, angels, spirit guides, plant and animal devas, crystal devas, fairies, other-planetary helpers, the Lords of Karma; puts one on the path to ascension or enlightenment. The Victorians used Oriental Poppies to denote silence; this essence reverses silence.

POPPY, Royal Wedding
(Papaver orientale)
(Crown) White

> **Add Gemstones:** White Apophyllite, Selenite, Angel Wing Selenite, Seraphanite, Phenacite, Diamond, Silver Aura Crystal, White Topaz, Clear Quartz Crystal, Danburite

> Develops and opens the crown chakra and entire kundalini line, clears and cleanses the crown and kundalini system, removes obstructions; rewires and repairs the crown chakra and crown complex (crown on all levels); heals core soul damage to the crown and crown complex, heals core soul damage to the kundalini line; repairs rips tears and holes in the aura and auric field, heals core soul damage to the aura; accelerates psychic opening, initiates and accelerates spiritual development and evolution, puts one on a direct and rapid path to ascension (enlightenment), removes and heals all that prevents spiritual enlightenment. The Victorians used this flower to symbolize sleep; the essence is for transcendence.

POPPY, Ruffled Patty

(Papaver orientale)

(Heart) Pink

> **Add Gemstones:** Spirit Quartz, Pink Druzy Quartz, Pink Sapphire, Pink Tourmaline, Watermelon Tourmaline, Lepidolite with Rubellite, Pink Calcite, Clear Quartz Crystal, Danburite
>
> Repairs and opens the heart chakra and heart complex (heart on all levels), repairs and opens the emotional body and hara line chakras and channels; heals and removes obstructions, rewires and repatterns; heals core soul damage of the heart, heart complex, hara line and emotional body; provides karmic release, grace and healing for past life suffering and heart center damage; removes all that prevents an open healed heart, promotes unconditional love, initiates forgiveness of oneself and all others; puts one on an evolutionary spiritual path, heals grief especially grief carried forward from other lifetimes

PORTULACA

(Portulaca grandiflora)

(Belly, Solar Plexus and Heart) Mixed Colors

> **Add Gemstones:** Garnet, Orange Calcite, Honey Calcite, Golden Topaz, Green Calcite, Pink Calcite, Rose Quartz, Amethyst, Phenacite, Clear Quartz Crystal, Danburite
>
> Brings laughter and joy back into one's life after grief and disappointment, heals traumas and difficult transitions, soothes heartache, promotes opening to the gifts of life and Goddess, promotes appreciating the beauty of one's life and the Earth; changes grief, depression, guilt or self-blame into acceptance, provides validation and inner peace, soothes and eases

PORTULACA
(Portulaca grandiflora)

(Heart) Pink

> **Add Gemstones:** Mangano Calcite, Rose Quartz, Pink Smithsonite, Pink Kunzite, Pink Andean Opal, Rhodonite, Pink Sapphire, Pink Tourmaline, Clear Quartz Crystal, Danburite
>
> Aids and supports children in learning about the world, helps make going to school positive, aids children in making friends; promotes children's learning from plants, animals, stones and people; helps in dealing with hurts and traumas on all levels, protects innocence, cushions and eases the fears and sorrows of childhood; eases disappointment, soothes, calms, reassures

PORTULACA
(Portulaca grandiflora)

(Belly) Orange

> **Add Gemstones:** Orange Calcite, Carnelian, Peach Moonstone, Sunstone, Jacinth (Orange Sapphire), Red Phantom Calcite, Sponge Coral, Clear Quartz Crystal, Danburite
>
> Supports girls entering menarche (first menstruation) and adolescence; promotes accepting and appreciating one's body, encourages good self-image, encourages positive self-love, aids in developing healthy independence and self-respect; promotes joy in becoming a woman, inspires joy in being female; aids friendship between girls, encourages good relationships between girls and their mothers; assists in opening to and understanding early sexuality and sensuality, reduces fears of growing up

PORTULACA
(Portulaca grandiflora)

(Perineum) Red

> **Add Gemstones:** Moroccan Red Quartz, Garnet, Cuprite, Ruby, Star Ruby, Spinel, Amethyst with Hematite, Red Phantom Quartz, Clear Quartz Crystal, Danburite
>
> Cushions and heals the process of falling in love for the first time or repeatedly, reinforces self-love; promotes a sense of reality about the other, aids in recognizing real from wishful relationships, heals unrequited love; heals disappointment in first love, heals puppy love, promotes sexual responsibility; grounds love and relationship into earth plane reality

PORTULACA
(Portulaca grandiflora)

(Solar Plexus) Yellow

> **Add Gemstones:** Honey Calcite, Yellow Opal, Golden Labradorite, Amber, Golden Topaz, Yellow Jade, Citrine, Rutile Citrine, Clear Quartz Crystal, Danburite
>
> Calms and stabilizes the mind, calms the nonphysical mental bodies and levels, heals and purifies the mental body; promotes mental clarity, stimulates the intellect, aids ability to make clear choices and decisions; increases assimilation of ideas and information, enhances good study habits and learning, increases the ability to memorize information, aids all learning; mood raiser, stabilizes confusion, increases information retention, calms mental distress

POWDER PUFF
(Calliandra haematocephala)
(Perineum) Red

> **Add Gemstones:** Red Moroccan Quartz, Garnet, Ruby, Rhodonite, Black Tourmaline, Red Obsidian, Hematite, Black Kyanite, Clear Quartz Crystal, Danburite
>
> Offers help in accepting and respecting one's physical body and appearance, aids creating a positive self-image, increases respect for one's body; helps those who feel ugly or who are physically damaged, good for teenagers; creates an awareness that "you are Goddess" and therefore perfect, aids being in the body and accepting the present incarnation fully, promotes an awareness of the beauty of one's soul

PRICKLY PEAR
(Opuntia sp.)
(Hara) Yellow

> **Add Gemstones:** Amber, Yellow Opal, Dravite, Honey Calcite, Yellow Jade, Yellow Apatite, Yellow Sunstone, Golden Beryl, Clear Quartz Crystal, Danburite
>
> Encourages the feeling of having a place in the world and the right to be here, promotes taking one's place proudly, effects taking one's space proudly; promotes an understanding that your actions and life have consequence, that you are needed in this world, that your life and work change the world for the better and help others; encourages feeling wanted, inspires positive self-image, stabilizes and soothes; helpful in difficult adolescence, supports people with eating disorders, helps those who can't relax

PRINCESS FLOWER TREE
(Tibouchina semidecandra)

(Crown) Purple

> **Add Gemstones:** Ametrine, Amethyst, Purple Fluorite, Alexandrite, Purple Sapphire, Purple Kunzite, Clear Beryl, Clear Kunzite, Herkimer Diamond, Danburite
>
> Assists in opening to spirituality, promotes accepting and letting in spiritual energy; induces spiritual awakening in those ready and willing for it, aids in recognizing oneself as a spiritual Be-ing; increases one's connection with spiritual guides, angels, the Lords of Karma and other Light Be-ings; protects from entities and energies that are not of the Light; promotes trust in one's part and place in the universal plan, accelerates spiritual growth and one's progress on the path to enlightenment or ascension

QUEEN OF THE NIGHT
(Selenicereus grandiflora)

(Transpersonal Point) White

> **Add Gemstones:** White Sapphire, Clear Beryl, White Moonstone, Diamond, Rainbow Moonstone, White Opal, Fire Opal, Phenacite, Herkimer Diamond, Danburite
>
> Powerful essence for moon magick, increases one's connection with the Goddess and the Moon, helps moon rituals, aids in Drawing Down the Moon; good for all women's rituals, inspires rituals of love and pleasure, good Wiccan energy; promotes group energy, magick, meditation, psychic opening; also promotes love, lesbian love, spiritual love unions, sexuality and orgasm, tantric sex; supports nonphysical (astral) love and lovers. This plant blooms briefly and only once a year; make the essence at night under the Moon.

QUEEN SAGO PALM
(Cycas circinalis)
(Movement) Tan

Add Gemstones: Sammonite, Ammonite Fossil, Boulder Opal, Jasper (Brown, any variety), Bone Coral, Brown Agate, Brown Pietersite, Tiger Eye, Herkimer Diamond, Danburite

Promotes strength in adversity, aids moving forward on one's life path despite all obstacles, overcomes obstruction and interference from others, eases and loosens negative stubbornness and resistance in oneself, strengthens and heals one's desire and ability to accomplish tasks and succeed, increases endurance; aids the ability and determination to do what is right

RAIN LILY
— *See ZEPHYR LILY*

RAINBOW SHOWER TREE
(Cassia fistula x javanica)
(Heart) Peach and Gold

Add Gemstones: Natural Citrine, Peach Moonstone, Rhodochrosite, Amber, Yellow Sunstone, Peach Sunstone, Golden Labradorite, Golden Beryl, Herkimer Diamond, Danburite

An essence for women's healing, promotes healing the damage of being female; heals one's self-image and self-worth of misogyny, racism, ableism, fat oppression, homophobia; brings to women a sense of being part of the family of all women; aids in healing the Earth of the damage done to women, aids in healing the Earth of the ravages of war; promotes manifesting a healed planet in oneself and through one's heart. This tree is also called Rainbow Cassia

ROSE, Angel Face
(Rosa sp.)
(Heart) Lavender Pink

> **Add Gemstones:** Pink Kunzite, Lepidolite, Spirit Quartz, Rose Quartz, Gem Rose Quartz, Pink Tourmaline, Pink Fresh Water Pearl, Angel Wing Selenite, Herkimer Diamond, Danburite

> Increases awareness and understanding of the angelic realm and angelic presence in one's life, promotes contact with personal angelic guides and guardian angels, increases divine guidance from the angelic realm; brings access to divine grace, aids the ability to receive forgiveness and to forgive, fosters compassion, promotes universal love, encourages self-love, helps heart healing, provides inner peace

ROSE, Baby Blanket
(Rosa sp.)
(Heart) Pink

> **Add Gemstones:** Pink Kunzite, Purple Kunzite, Green Kunzite, Pink Sapphire, Morganite, Raspberry Garnet, Rose Quartz, Mangano Calcite, Herkimer Diamond, Danburite

> A flower energy primarily for babies and children; soothes, calms and protects, assists in adjusting to a new incarnation, eases fear and confusion; promotes the growth and development of the energy bodies and chakras on all levels, stabilizes the silver cord that connects life to the body; aids in resolving karmic issues between child and parent, helps the new mother and father to adjust to being parents, helps the child to feel loved and wanted; promotes curiosity and learning about life

ROSE, Bibi Maizoon
(Rosa sp.)
(Heart) Pink

> **Add Gemstones:** Gem Rose Quartz, Pink Sapphire, Gem Rhodochrosite, Pink Spirit Quartz, Lepidolite, Pink Druzy Quartz, Pink Tourmaline, Pink Kunzite, Herkimer Diamond, Danburite
>
> Stabilizes and heals the heart and emotions, heals the emotional body and inner child, promotes core soul heart healing on the kundalini level, offers heart chakra repair and rescue, heals in layers from the surface inward; promotes and aids deep emotional transformation and change, releases and heals heart scars gently; soothes, insulates and comforts, brings joy where there was none or little before; brings about "ah ha" moments of deep understanding and healing

ROSE, Brandy
(Rosa sp.)
(Belly) Yellow-Orange

> **Add Gemstones:** Peach Moonstone, Peach Aventurine, Mexican Opal, Jelly Opal, Peach Calcite, Honey Calcite, Amber, Clear Quartz Crystal, Danburite
>
> Cleanses, clears, protects and heals the belly chakra and emotional body; aids in releasing pictures of past traumas and abuse from this life and past lives that are held in the belly chakra; heals the inner child, provides emotional reprogramming for recovery from abuse; promotes soul retrieval and healing of soul fragments (finds, brings in, heals and reintegrates soul fragments); promotes core soul healing especially of the emotional levels, provides emotional soothing and protection for those doing difficult emotional work

ROSE, Charlotte
(Rosa sp.)

(Solar Plexus) Yellow

> **Add Gemstones:** Yellow Kyanite, Amber, Tiger Eye, Citrine, Yellow Topaz, Champagne Topaz, Lemon Yellow Calcite, Golden Beryl, Herkimer Diamond, Danburite
>
> Cleanses, clears and detoxifies the emotions and emotional body, shields and protects the emotional body; removes and destroys negative cords and hooks that connect to others from this or other lifetimes, prevents removed cords and hooks from being reattached; provides protection from needy and grasping people who are emotionally or psychically draining (called psychic vampires), good protection for healers and social workers; helps to balance one's energy during detoxification processes

ROSE—CLIMBING, Amadeus
(Rosa sp.)

(Root) Red

> **Add Gemstones:** Garnet, White Moonstone, Selenite, White Fresh Water Pearl, Mother of Pearl, White Opal, Fire Opal, Herkimer Diamond, Danburite
>
> An essence for young girls approaching womanhood; promotes and eases changes and transitions, supports the firsts in a girl's life; facilitates menarche (first menstruation), balances the excitement of first dates and first love, supports adolescents and young women; protects girls' innocence and supports maturing awareness; sustains through all the adolescent rites of passage, turns transformation into blooming

ROSE—CLIMBING, Cinderella
(Rosa sp.)
(Heart) Pink

Add Gemstone: Pink Druzy Quartz, Pink Fluorite, Lepido-lite with Mica, Rose Quartz, Peach Moonstone, Pink Andean Opal, Pink Kunzite, Herkimer Diamond, Danburite

An essence for toddlers and children; insulates and soothes situations of change, transition, growth and transformation; cushions changing from toddler to child and child to preteen; protects innocence and helps maturing; helps in understand-ing and learning to live successfully in the world; assists in making first friends and first best friends; helps with adjusting to school or daycare; supports all the firsts of childhood

ROSE, Dainty Bess
(Rosa sp.)
(Heart) Pink

Add Gemstones: Pink Kunzite, Rose Quartz, Rhodochrosite, Pink Calcite, Mangano Calcite, Rhodonite, Pink Andean Opal, Raspberry Garnet, Herkimer Diamond, Danburite

Heals damage to the creational Moment of Self and all heart systems and connections (the heart complex and more); sup-ports and promotes personal freedom and independence, helps those who are codependent or needy to strengthen their resolve, promotes personal independent strength, aids becoming a strong and independent person, creates self-suffi-ciency in those lacking it or just growing into it; good essence for women in recovery or who have survived abuse

ROSE, Desert Peace
(Rosa sp.)

(Hara) Yellow and Red

> **Add Gemstones:** Spinel, Garnet, Rhodochrosite, Golden Labradorite, Golden Beryl, Ruby, Star Ruby, Amber, Golden Topaz, Herkimer Diamond, Danburite
>
> Promotes walking in peace on Mother Earth, encourages living consciously with nature; creates inner peace, enhances the concept of "being peace" by one's living example, aids being peaceful in oneself and in all dealings with others; fosters awareness of the oneness of all that lives, fosters compassion; provides certainty of one's life path, aids knowing who you are and why you are here, aids seeing the self as Goddess; an all-healing essence with the focus on peace; calms and soothes

ROSE, Double Delight
(Rosa sp.)

(Crown and Root) Red and White

> **Add Gemstones:** Ruby, Star Ruby, Black Star Sapphire, Garnet, Diamond, Chrysanthemum Stone, Selenite, Amethyst with Hematite, Ruby with Zoisite, Clear Quartz Crystal, Danburite
>
> Spiritualizes love and passion, promotes union between true lovers, aids in building a life and relationship together; supports marriage and daily life, promotes passionate sexuality as expressions of real love; supports gay, lesbian and heterosexual love and union; promotes joy in each other, increases harmony together, inspires seeing oneself and one's mate as Goddess or God; brings soul mates and twin flames together and supports their spiritual union on Earth

ROSE, Garden Party
(Rosa sp.)
(Crown) Cream White

> **Add Gemstones:** Champagne Topaz, Amber, Smoky Quartz, White Opal, Dravite (Golden Tourmaline), Clear Kunzite, Clear Beryl, Golden Beryl, Clear Quartz Crystal, Danburite
>
> Heals and balances all the kundalini line chakras and energy flows, fills the aura with Light and healing; soothes, balances and stabilizes all aura energy and the entire auric envelope; provides a sense of emotional security and being fully loved by other people and the Goddess, promotes trust in the universe and in the processes of life; aids life transitions, promotes universal and unconditional love

ROSE, Gold Badge
(Rosa sp.)
(Solar Plexus) Yellow

> **Add Gemstones:** Tiger Eye, Amber, Natural Citrine, Dravite (Golden Tourmaline), Topaz, Yellow Fluorite, Yellow Calcite, Yellow Jade, Clear Quartz Crystal, Danburite
>
> Provides energy balancing and alignment of the energy bodies and chakras; removes energy blockages and obstructions, cleanses the energy systems of negative entities and attacks; provides all-aura protection and general psychic protection, operates as a psychic shield, heals exposure to negative energies and interference; protects from being controlled by others and from the tendency to control others, promotes right use of will; fills the aura with Light, provides peace and healing

ROSE, Gypsy Carnival
(Rosa sp.)

(Root) Red and Yellow

> **Add Gemstones:** Hessionite Garnet, Yellow Opal, Amber, Yellow Topaz, Red Garnet, Ruby, Spinel, Moroccan Red Quartz, Clear Quartz Crystal, Danburite
>
> Promotes love and healing, supports healing through sexual love and the loving expression of sexuality; establishes the relationship polarity of those alike and opposite (heterosexual love, homosexual love); supports sexuality as a healing aspect of relationship stability, affirms marriage or sexual union, aids in expressing the joy of responsible passion, promotes joyful love and lovers

ROSE, Lagerfeld
(Rosa sp.)

(Causal Body) Lavender Pink

> **Add Gemstones:** Lepidolite, Purple Kunzite, Pink Kunzite, Blue Kunzite, Pink Sapphire, Pink Tourmaline, Violet Tourmaline, Rose Quartz, Gem Rose Quartz, Herkimer Diamond, Danburite
>
> Provides emotional aid, comfort, rescue, safety, security, peace of mind and soul; encourages awareness of the oneness of all life, a reminder of every individual's oneness with the Goddess and that everyone carries the Goddess within them, helps in understanding one's place and part in the wholeness of life; provides pain relief, eases fear and panic, eases depression and anxiety; helps in times of trauma, turmoil, overwhelm, terror and crisis

ROSE, Lasting Peace
(Rosa sp.)
(Belly) Orange

> **Add Gemstones:** Red Jasper, Carnelian, Vanadinite, Honey Calcite, Mexican Opal, Jelly Opal, Selenite, Diamond, Herkimer Diamond, Danburite
>
> Promotes peace, prosperity and plenty in one's life; aids all aspects of material stability, supports stable marriage or long term relationships; provides certainty of one's place and path on Earth, encourages knowledge of being wanted and needed and that one's work and life have consequence, supports making the world a better place by your actions and life, supports making your life whole and loving; promotes women's menstrual balance and fertility, warms and fills with love

ROSE, Medallion
(Rosa sp.)
(Hara) Peach

> **Add Gemstones:** Peach Calcite, Feldspar, Mexican Opal, Pecos Diamond (Orange Quartz), Peach Sunstone, Peach Aventurine, Peach Moonstone, Jelly Opal, Herkimer Diamond, Danburite
>
> Safely heals anger from this life and past lives, releases karmic anger patterns, changes self-anger to self-love, supports the healing of those who express anger in self-defeating ways; frees one to find and accomplish one's life purpose and reason for incarnating; balances the hara line and hara chakras; eases depression, encourages and increases self-empowerment

ROSE—MINIATURE, Child's Play

(Heart) Pink

> **Add Gemstones:** Gem Rose Quartz, Mangano Calcite, Pink Calcite, Rhodochrosite, Pink Chinese Opal, Pink Andean Opal, Herkimer Diamond, Danburite
>
> Provides soothing emotional healing for women, children and pets; all animal healing but especially useful for cats; calms, brings confidence in being loved; promotes joy, music and ritual; opens the heart to receiving joy, heals grief, lifts depression, reduces fear, promotes creativity and trust

ROSE—MINIATURE, Rainbow's End

(Rosa sp.)

(Hara) Red and Yellow

> **Add Gemstones:** Agate—Multi Mixed Colors, Mookite, Red Jasper, Yellow Jasper, Yellow Jade, Amber, Garnet, Phenacite, Clear Quartz Crystal, Danburite
>
> Increases connection to the angelic realm, helps in working with the angels for Earth healing; offers protection and guidance for those who bring cosmic information to Earth understanding, helps in channeling information from the angels for use in planetary evolution; offers angelic healing for the Earth and its caretakers; provides angelic protection from evil and attack

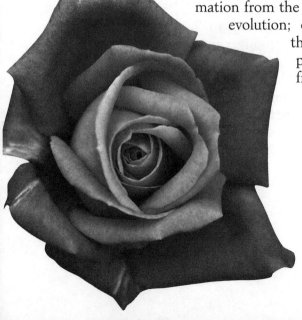

ROSE—MINIATURE, Starina
(Rosa sp.)

(Perinium) Red

> **Add Gemstones:** Red Tiger Eye, Red Pietersite, Moroccan Red Quartz, Cuprite, Garnet, Ruby, Star Ruby, Red Spinel, Phenacite, Clear Quartz Crystal, Danburite

> Brings wisdom to the Earth and Earth living, promotes living wisely and walking gently and with passion on the planet, aids in applying spiritual knowledge and information to real life problems and situations, promotes living in the present and being here now, uses practical knowledge to promote wellness and well-being, heals the body-mind connection, aids grounding

ROSE, Oregold
(Rosa sp.)

(Solar Plexus) Yellow

> **Add Gemstones:** Tiger Eye, Amber, Yellow Opal, Yellow Jade, Golden Topaz, Golden Beryl, Yellow Fluorite, Golden Labradorite, Natural Citrine, Herkimer Diamond, Danburite

> Radiates a rainbow energy that cleanses, clears, calms and balances all the kundalini chakras; supports life transitions and completions, promotes stability and inner peace after a process of change, provides equilibrium; aids recognition of new inner growth, aids self-validation of work well done; supports healthy self-esteem, joyful and warming, brings in Light

ROSE, Pascali
(Rosa sp.)

(Transpersonal Point) White

> **Add Gemstones:** Selenite, Phenacite, White Moonstone, Rainbow Moonstone, Fire Opal, Clear Beryl, Clear Kunzite, Clear Fluorite, Herkimer Diamond, Danburite
>
> For love and union, promotes and encourages a true soul mate union of body and soul, spiritualizes love, releases and heals karma between soul mates that would impede or prevent a perfect union; promotes total trust and unconditional love between oneself and the beloved; provides high level core soul healing of all damage from this and past lifetimes; repairs soul fragmentation—heals, brings in and integrates fragmented soul parts, facilitates soul retrieval work; repairs the DNA; promotes connection with Goddess, fills the aura and all bodies with Light and love; provides inner peace, all-healing

ROSE, Peace
(Rosa sp.)

(Hara) Pink and Yellow

> **Add Gemstones:** Yellow Opal, Amber, Rose Quartz, Rutile Citrine, Pink Tourmaline, Pink Sapphire, Lepidolite with Mica, Kunzite (any color), Herkimer Diamond, Danburite
>
> Heals and balances all of the hara line chakras and energy flows, stabilizes the kundalini heart chakra and entire heart complex (heart on all levels); fills the aura with Light and healing; stabilizes during processes of intense change, supports life transitions and deep healing, promotes all healing including core soul healing; gives a sense of courage, strength and security during energy shifts; helps to prepare one for change, increases trust in change and in life's processes; soothes and eases trauma, stress and transformation. Called Rose of the Century, this is the most popular rose in floral history.

ROSE, Perfume Beauty
(Rosa sp.)
(Heart) Pink

> **Add Gemstones:** Pink Druzy Quartz, Spirit Quartz, Pink Tourmaline, Lepidolite, Pink Kunzite, Morganite, Pink Smithsonite, Rose Aura Crystal, Clear Quartz Crystal, Danburite
>
> For attracting and sustaining love and union, promotes the union of body and soul, attracts soul mate relationships, promotes deep mutual love and openness between partners; increases empathy, fosters caring, encourages unconditional love, promotes fidelity, supports trust; helps to create a marriage of true minds and hearts, helps to form harmonious and peaceful relationships, begins lifelong relationships, finds true love

ROSE, Playboy
(Rosa sp.)
(Hara) Peach and Gold

> **Add Gemstones:** Mexican Opal, Jelly Opal, Peach Moonstone, Peach Calcite, Orange Garnet, Orange Sapphire, Yellow Opal, Yellow Sapphire, Clear Quartz Crystal, Danburite
>
> Brings relaxation and play into one's life, provides a time-out from work and worry, heals the inner child; helps to heal burnout, aids the workaholic in slowing down; reduces fear of joblessness, emotionally assists those looking for work, assists those whose jobs are abhorrent to them; eases insecurity, reduces feeling not good enough; assists grief recovery, promotes hope, increases optimism, inspires joy, fosters inner peace

ROSE, Princess of Monaco
(Rosa sp.)

(Heart) Pink and White

> **Add Gemstones:** Watermelon Tourmaline, Pink Sapphire, Gem Rose Quartz, Gem Rhodochrosite, Pink Kunzite, Golden Amber, Pink Tourmaline, Herkimer Diamond, Danburite
>
> For all-aura calming and stabilizing, heals and balances the entire hara and kundalini lines, a powerful emotional rescue essence; helps in times of shock, fear, trauma, stress or pain; aids the ability to keep one's heart open during stress, promotes the ability to function well during emergency situations of one's own or others'; a useful energy for adults, children, infants, pets; soothes, calms, fosters clarity of mind and rapid good decisions

ROSE, Queen Elizabeth
(Rosa sp.)

(Heart) Pink

> **Add Gemstones:** Rose Aura Crystal, Mangano Calcite, Pink Kunzite, Gem Rose Quartz, Lepidolite with Mica, Morganite, Pink Andean Opal, Pink Coral, Pink Sapphire, Herkimer Diamond, Danburite
>
> Promotes positive self-image, strong self-esteem and self-worth, positive self-love, solid self-confidence; provides calm and emotional balance, encourages inner peace; supports a balanced ability to give and receive, promotes compassion and forgiveness of oneself and others; draws love and unconditional love; a good essence for girls, adolescents, and women, especially helpful for women in recovery; heals the emotions and the heart

ROSE, Redgold
(Rosa sp.)

(Solar Plexus) Fuschia and Gold

> **Add Gemstones:** Rhodochrosite, Rhodonite, Raspberry Garnet, Red Pietersite, Amber, Yellow Kyanite, Amber Calcite, Citrine, Clear Quartz Crystal, Danburite
>
> Balances will with compassion and aids in putting compassion first; promotes trust in life and the Goddess; aids learning to let go, encourages the ability to surrender the mind to the heart and soul; encourages opening oneself to honest emotion and feeling; supports mental and emotional stability, offers inner peace

ROSE, Reine des violettes
(Rosa sp.)

(Crown) Violet

> **Add Gemstones:** Amethyst, Canadian Amethyst, Purple Fluorite, Sugilite, Pink Tourmaline, Violet Tourmaline, Purple Fluorite, Moldavite, Herkimer Diamond, Danburite
>
> Opens and clears the kundalini and hara line channels and chakras, removes energy blockages and obstructions to energy flows and movement; clears negative interference including alien implants, releases possessions and negative entities, ends psychic attacks; accesses positive intergalactic healers and helpers for protection from interference and attack, protects and guards

ROSE, Royal Velvet
(Rosa sp.)
(Perineum) Red

> **Add Gemstones:** Black Opal, Garnet, Black Kyanite, Tektite, Red Coral, Spinel, Ruby, Black Tourmaline, Black Velvet Tourmaline, Clear Quartz Crystal, Danburite
>
> Grounds and roots the incarnation and one's life purpose into the earth plane, heals and attaches one's connection (grounding cord) fully to the planet; a good flower essence for those with a strong life purpose of service to the Earth and people as well as for those who are not enough following their life purpose; makes one aware of their life path and intensifies the will to accomplish it; aids those who are peaceful destroyers of evil and injustice, promotes clear intent, increases courage, inspires one to protect all goodness and truth; offers psychic protection

ROSE, Sonia
(Rosa sp.)
(Heart) Salmon Pink

> **Add Gemstones:** Dolomite, Lepidolite, Pink Sapphire, Raspberry Garnet, Pink Calcite, Pink Tourmaline, Kunzite, Pink Coral, Herkimer Diamond, Danburite
>
> For repairing and healing the emotional heart and emotional body, heals the heart chakra on all levels (heart complex), releases heart scars by dissolving them gently; heals long term emotional pain and despair, heals karmic pain; soothes and heals grief, eases loneliness, reduces feeling helpless, ends hopelessness; provides comfort, inspires hope, affords patience, encourages forgiveness; encourages universal and unconditional love for others and oneself

ROSE, Spice Twice
(Rosa sp.)
(Belly) Orange and White

> **Add Gemstones:** Carnelian, Vanadinite, Selenite, Orange Calcite, Golden Selenite, Jacinth (Orange Sapphire), Jelly Opal, Herkimer Diamond, Danburite
>
> Promotes putting the spice back in one's life, accelerates emotional healing and the return of joy; increases the will to live, encourages the desire for each new day's experiences, increases a sense of wellness and well-being; supports healing and recovery after surgery or emotional loss, promotes healing from shock and trauma of all kinds; aids emotional recovery after abortion or miscarriage, heals after relationship breakups, promotes sexual healing; gives one the will to continue and prevail

ROSE, Summer Fashion
(Rosa sp.)
(Heart) Pink and Yellow

> **Add Gemstones:** Rose Aura Crystal, Mangano Calcite, Pink Calcite, Amber, Rose Quartz, Pink Kunzite, Morganite, Clear Quartz Crystal, Danburite
>
> Heals the transition and trauma of birth and entering the world, aids new mothers and babies, aids infants' adaptation to living in a body, helps threatened infants to decide to stay on Earth, facilitates full connection of the soul to the body; helps an infant or child to feel secure and safe, promotes feeling welcome and wanted, increases a child's awareness of being loved; use as an infant and children's rescue essence that is also for insecure new mothers

ROSE, Tropicana
(Rosa sp.)
(Belly) Orange

> **Add Gemstones:** Vanadinite, Carnelian, Carnelian Agate, Jacinth (Orange Sapphire), Orange Calcite, Pecos Quartz (Pecos Diamond), Jelly Opal, Mexican Opal, Clear Quartz Crystal, Danburite

> Emotionally rebalances women's reproductive systems after trauma; heals the entire kundalini and hara line systems, promotes core soul healing with regard to reproductive and sexual karma, aids in karmic release for these issues; provides emotional assistance to women who have been battered or raped, supports after hysterectomy or other reproductive surgery; aids emotional recovery after abortion, helps women adjust to menopause

ROSE, Wild Climbing Tea
(Rosa sp.)
(Heart) Pink

> **Add Gemstones:** Rose Quartz, Watermelon Tourmaline, Rose Aura Crystal, Peach Moonstone, Pink Calcite, Pink Coral, Rainbow Moonstone, Herkimer Diamond, Danburite

> Helps one to heal and learn from the past (this life and past incarnations), aids in remembering past lives, helps in perceiving and releasing negative karmic patterns, helps to bring what was good in the past to operate again in the present, brings the good old days into now; heals heart scars gently, assists emotional body healing, helps to heal the heart, changes sorrow into quiet joy, promotes trust and acceptance

ROSE, Winchester Cathedral

(Transpersonal Point) White

> **Add Gemstones:** White Moonstone, Angel Wing Selenite, White Opal, Rainbow Moonstone, Phenacite, White Chalcedony, White Apophyllite, Herkimer Diamond, Danburite
>
> Repairs, cleanses, opens and clears the Transpersonal Point chakra (the emotional body, hara line crown chakra); heals the emotional body and all hara line channels and chakras; clears, heals and cleanses the templates (the doorways between bodies); fills the energy channels with Light, prepares to anchor the Higher Self into the body (brings the soul into the body); aids core soul healing, repairs the DNA, initiates and promotes all ascension and enlightenment processes and preparations

ROSE MALLOW

(Hibiscus moscheuto)

(Heart) Mixed Colors—pink, white, red

> **Add Gemstones:** Aqua Aura Crystal, Rose Aura Crystal, Silver Aura Crystal, Opal Aura Crystal, Rose Quartz, Gem Rose Quartz, Phenacite, Herkimer Diamond, Danburite
>
> Assists in new beginnings and healthy relationships after recovery from past relationship abuse; return hope, ability to trust, ability for heart opening, completes the grief process; supports a positive and joyful life after trauma, incest, rape, battering, war, cancer, hysterectomy or breast removal; heals and repairs the emotional and other energy bodies, heals the kundalini line chakras and channels; supports going forward with joy

ROSE MALLOW
(Hibiscus moscheuto)
(Thymus) White

> **Add Gemstones:** Aqua Aura Crystal, Silver Aura Crystal, Opal Aura Crystal, Eilat Stone, Gem Silica, Amazonite, Turquoise, Blue Andean Opal, Phenacite, Herkimer Diamond, Danburite
>
> Promotes recovery and healing from past abuse, facilitates grief recovery, aids forgiveness of others and oneself, releases guilt and blame, eases self-blame, reduces resentment; helps to heal the emotional body, astral body, hara line chakras and channels, inner child and higher self; aids in rebuilding a positive and joyful life after incest, rape, battering; helps with emotional recovery after hysterectomy or breast surgery, offers emotional support for the immune system

ROSE OF SHARON
(Hibiscus syriacus)
(Third Eye) Blue

> **Add Gemstones:** Azurite, Blue Aventurine, Blue Labradorite, Blue Quartz, Angelite, Blue Sapphire, Blue Tourmaline, Sodalite, Lapis Lazuli, Clear Quartz Crystal, Danburite
>
> Clears the third eye (Kundalini line) and vision chakras (hara line); opens one to psychic seeing and knowing, promotes clairvoyance and other psychic visual skills (crystal gazing, visualization, psychic healing); promotes contact with positive alien Light Be-ings; increases contact with nonphysical teachers, healers, Earth healers and helpers; promotes contact with spirit guides, angels, fairies, devas, and Be-ings from other dimensions and realms; initiates and aids spiritual growth and understanding, offers mind expansion, reprograms the mind grid, facilitates karmic healing and reprogramming

SAGE, Mexican Blue
(Salvia hispanica)
(Throat) Blue

> **Add Gemstones:** Holly Blue Agate, Celestite, Blue Lace Agate, Blue Druzy Chalcedony, Blue Labradorite, Blue Sapphire, Blue Dumortierite, Herkimer Diamond, Danburite
>
> Heals the voice and throat, clears and removes obstructions and blockages to one's ability for free expression, heals one's ability to express personal and spiritual truths; promotes the ability to speak out and speak one's objections, outrage and needs; ends the destructive keeping in of secrets and shame; releases karmic constrictions of throat and voice, releases and destroys negative attachments and entities; clears the throat chakra and throat complex (throat on all levels); promotes psychic expressions like channeling, supports teaching and singing, heals all expressions of creativity

SAGE, White
(Salvia apiana)
(Throat) Blue

> **Add Gemstones:** Azurite, Blue Dumortierite, Lapis Lazuli, Blue Aventurine, Blue Sapphire, Blue Tourmaline, Celestite, Clear Quartz Crystal, Danburite
>
> For the throat and voice, opens and stabilizes self-expression and all creativity—singing, speaking, acting, writing, art; promotes speaking one's truth, encourages expressing one's needs and wants; helps in overcoming fear, increases honesty, encourages honor, supports courage, helps with tact and wisdom; reduces stage fright and shyness, reduces being tongue-tied, releases the lump in the throat from needful things unsaid; helps women who have been told all their lives to "shut up and be quiet"

SEA OATS
(Chasmanthium sp.)

(Movement) Green and Tan

Add Gemstones: Serpentine Jade, Ocean Jasper, Picture Jasper, Boulder Opal, Moldavite, Bone Coral, Pietersite, Rainforest Jasper, Herkimer Diamond, Danburite

Promotes attunement to the sea; initiates contact with sea spirits and sea Goddesses, whales and dolphins, sea turtles, manatees, sea birds, mythological sea creatures and mermaids; supports and balances body rhythms and moon cycles, promotes understanding the cycles of evolution and of life; provides healing for the emotional body and the kundalini chakras; supports women's cycles of fertility, menstruation and menopause; cleanses and calms. Sea Oats are a protected plant in many beach locations and it may be illegal to pick them.

SHRIMP PLANT
(Justicia Brandegeana)

(Movement) Bronze

Add Gemstones: Pietersite, Green Tourmaline, Emerald, Moldavite, Sammonite, Boulder Opal, Brown Jasper, Green Amber, Green Zincite, Clear Quartz Crystal, Danburite

Promotes joyful movement forward on one's life path, helps in knowing one's life purpose and having the ability to achieve it, creates joy and pride in one's purpose and accomplishment, promotes steady progress toward life goals; aids in finding guidance on one's path, protects from delay and negativity, overcomes adversity and obstruction; an essence for the Goddess Green Tara. Two Latin names are listed for the Shrimp plant and used interchangeably—Beloperone gutatta and Justicia brandegeana.

SHRIMP PLANT
(Justicia brandegeana)
(Heart) Pink

> **Add Gemstones:** Pink Druzy Quartz, Spirit Quartz, Rose Quartz, Rose Aura Crystal, Mangano Calcite, Watermelon Tourmaline, Pink Tourmaline, Pink Kunzite, Herkimer Diamond, Danburite
>
> Causes the heart to bloom with joy and love, heals the heart and heart complex (all levels of the heart), dissolves heart scars gently; heals heartache, grief, heartbreak, lost love, emotional trauma, loneliness, disappointment; promotes heart opening and the ability to receive love and feel joy, inspires forgiveness for oneself and all others, inspires unconditional love; for all heart healing

SHRIMP PLANT
(Beloperone guttata)
(Transpersonal Point) White

> **Add Gemstones:** Silver Aura Crystal, White Moonstone, Diamond, Clear Beryl, Angel Wing Selenite, Snow Quartz, Phenacite, Clear Quartz Crystal, Danburite
>
> Balances all the kundalini chakras and the full aura; eases kundalini rising and psychic opening, eases too rapid psychic development, soothes transition states; repairs and heals the higher energy bodies, promotes core soul cleansing and healing; reduces negativity and negative interference, repairs damage to the DNA from interference; promotes spiritual evolution by keeping it comfortable and safe, promotes transformation

SHRIMP PLANT
(Pachystachys lutea)

(Solar Plexus) Yellow

> **Add Gemstones:** Golden Topaz, Golden Beryl, Yellow Opal, Yellow Jade, Yellow Jasper, Amber, Natural Citrine, Lemon Yellow Calcite, Clear Quartz Crystal, Danburite
>
> Supports a healthy and uninflated self-image; fosters positive pride, promotes acceptance of self, encourages honest self-validation, fosters positive body image, increases low self-confidence; helps those who have lost breasts or other body parts to accept their bodies; cleanses and clears, purifies, fills with Light; aids in finding one's angels and one's wings; mood raising and calming; can be used in a sprayer to clear crystals

SILK OAK TREE
(Grevillea robusta)

(Hara) Orange

> **Add Gemstones:** Amber, Champagne Topaz, Jacinth (Orange Sapphire), Red Jasper, Orange Garnet, Orange Zincite, Honey Calcite, Herkimer Diamond, Danburite
>
> Develops and opens the hara line chakras and channels, works to cleanse and purify the entire hara line and emotional body, heals and repairs; helps in finding and identifying one's life purpose and aids beginning to manifest it; supports beginning sexual opening, shields first sexual experiences and love affairs; increases wanting to be alive, promotes independent living

SKY VINE
(Thunbergia grandiflora)
(Throat) Blue

> **Add Gemstones:** Blue Sapphire, Angelite, Blue Aventurine, Azurite, Blue Druzy Chalcedony, Blue Opal, Blue Tourmaline, Iolite, Herkimer Diamond, Danburite
>
> An essence for all-healing, especially useful for healers and Earth healers; provides gentle transformation and positive change, supports all life changes; creates peace of mind, happiness, creativity, self-expression, aids in expressing one's truths, promotes spiritual growth and evolution; increases psychic abilities for channeling and psychic healing, increases one's contact with the planet for planetary healing; aids contact with spirit guides and angels, increases contact with the Goddess and understanding of the Goddess within

SKY VINE
(Thunbergia sp.)
(Belly) Peach

> **Add Gemstones:** Peach Moonstone, Carnelian, Amber, Amber Calcite, Peach Aventurine, Mexican Opal, Jelly Opal, Pink Andean Opal, Herkimer Diamond, Danburite
>
> General all-healer, supports every kind of healing by the strengthening of all nonphysical systems and anatomy; promotes emotional healing, aids regeneration and recovery from emotional or physical trauma, supports healing after surgery or illness; provides emotional support for healers, prevents and heals burnout and exhaustion; enables easier relaxation and rest

SKY VINE
(Thunbergia alata)

(Transpersonal Point) White

> **Add Gemstones:** Silver Aura Crystal, Opal Aura Crystal, Phenacite, White Moonstone, Fresh Water Pearl, Angel Wing Selenite, Herkimer Diamond, Danburite
>
> Draws in energy, healing and unconditional love from the angelic realm, promotes connection with angels and finding your guardian angel, increases understanding of the angelic realm, aids channeling angel energy and creativity; increases knowledge of the soul, promotes soul level healing and all healing; transforms negative karma, promotes DNA connection and healing, promotes spiritual evolution

SKY VINE
(Thunbergia grandaflora)

(Crown) White

> **Add Gemstones:** White Sapphire, White Phantom Quartz, White Moonstone, Phenacite, Selenite, Clear Beryl, Clear Kunzite, White Jade, Herkimer Diamond, Danburite
>
> Stimulates transformation in one's life and on the planet, triggers revelations and "ah ha" moments that change one's life; promotes and catalyses needed change, pushes those who procrastinate or are stuck, initiates spiritual awakening; promotes life changing experiences that can't be ignored; makes needed things happen in and around you; provides stability during personal and planetary changes, good essence for those who's work is planetary healing

SPATHYPHYLLUM
—See WHITE FLAG

SPIDER LILY
(Lycoris aurea)
(Hara) Orange and Yellow

Add Gemstones: Peach Sunstone, Yellow Sunstone, Amber, Red Jasper, Dravite (Golden Tourmaline), Champagne Topaz, Orange Zincite, Honey Calcite, Clear Quartz Crystal, Danburite

Stimulates creativity and inspiration in accordance with one's life purpose, offers the certainty and energy to manifest one's life purpose on the earth plane; promotes calm intent, determination, aids the ability to stay on one's karmic path, manifests karmic rewards and gifts; increases joy in one's life and in following one's life purpose, helps in making one's life purpose into one's livelihood

SPIDER LILY
(lycoris radiata)
(Belly) Red and Orange

Add Gemstones: Red Jasper, Red Coral, Moroccan Red Quartz, Gem Rhodochrosite, Spinel, Honey Calcite, Red Pietersite, Red Tiger Eye, Clear Quartz Crystal, Danburite

For creation of new life, new ideas or new art; promotes all creativity and all inspiration, aids new starts, establishes new projects, opens artist's block, heals procrastination; inspires fertility of mind and body, encourages conception; aids the ability to visualize and to use visualization as a tool, stores the pictures of what you wish to manifest, aids manifesting and bringing the pictures into physical reality

SPIDER LILY
(Hymenocallis sp.)
(Throat) White

> **Add Gemstones:** Gem Silica, Larimar, Blue Opal, Blue Calcite, Blue Lace Agate, Blue Coral, Blue Tourmaline, Turquoise, Blue Fluorite, Herkimer Diamond, Danburite
>
> Stimulates creativity, encourages free expression, fosters artistry, helps singing, promotes inspiration; opens artist's block, especially useful for singers and musicians but aids in all artistic expression; increases connection with spirit guides, muses, angelic realm, and the Goddess; a helpful essence for channelers and to use in channeling sessions; reduces stress, increases concentration, stimulates psychic abilities, calms

STEPHANOTIS
(Stephanotis jasminoides)
(Transpersonal Point) White

> **Add Gemstones:** Phenacite, Chrysoprase, Emerald, Dioptase, Diopside, Green Aventurine, True Jade, Green Serpentine Jade, Clear Quartz Crystal, Danburite
>
> Provides calm and balance during transitions, eases change and transformation; supports all physical, emotional, mental and spiritual practices and healing; aids mental and karmic repatterning, deepens karmic healing and release; promotes core soul healing and eases the process, promotes healing of all kinds; supports all spirituality; soothes, insulates, comforts. Also called Wedding Jasmine or Madagascar Jasmine; frequently used for bridal wreaths. Interestingly, the flower has the Victorian message of boasting too much!

SUNFLOWER, Giant
(Helianthus sp.)

(Hara) Yellow and Brown

> **Add Gemstones:** Sunstone, Amber, Amber Calcite, Topaz, Gold Fluorite, Brown Jasper, Mookite, Boulder Opal, Tiger Eye, Clear Quartz Crystal, Danburite
>
> Encourages a balance of body and spirit; promotes manifesting, abundance, prosperity, success; encourages self-confidence, honesty, good health; helps in finding and achieving one's life purpose, aids in turning one's avocation into one's joyful vocation, inspires and aids in making a contribution to help the world; helps in being financially successful without greed and with wise use of wealth, promotes generosity and giving; promotes joyful living, accomplishment, fulfillment, achievement with pleasure and joy

SWEET PEA
(Lathyrus odoratus)

(Crown) Lavender

> **Add Gemstones:** Sugilite, Lepidolite, Canadian Amethyst, Rose Quartz, Charoite, Violet Tourmaline, Purple Sapphire, Clear Quartz Crystal, Danburite
>
> Encourages recognizing and appreciating the sweetness of life, aids in tempering sadness with joy; promotes spiritual certainty and security; increases connection with and trust in Goddess and the Light, increases the ability to "let go and let Goddess"; eases fears and nightmares, promotes restful sleep, calms and soothes. In the flower language, sweet peas connote delicate pleasures and departures.

SWEET PEA
(Lathyrus odoratus)

(Perineum) Red

> **Add Gemstones:** Red Tiger Eye, Star Ruby, Garnet, Spinel, Red Coral, Labradorite, Rainbow Moonstone, Silver Aura Crystal, Phenacite, Herkimer Diamond, Danburite
>
> Brings one's life purpose into conscious awareness, facilitates the ways and means of achieving and manifesting one's life plan, increases the desire to achieve one's life path; promotes consciousness of other realms and dimensions, aids in transmitting and receiving conscious psychic information from positive other-planetary helpers and healers, aids channeling of ascended spiritual Be-ings

SWEET PEA
(Lathrus Odoratus)

(All Chakras) Multi Colors—White, Red, Pink, Lavender, Yellow used together

> **Add Gemstones:** Opal Aura Crystal, Cuprite, Rainbow Moonstone, Rose Aura Crystal, Aqua Aura Crystal, Green Kunzite, Purple Kunzite, Yellow Opal, Amber, Clear Quartz Crystal, Danburite
>
> Assists in chakra opening, chakra stabilizing and energy balancing for the entire kundalini line; promotes opening to the joy and sweetness in one's life and in all life; encourages an open heart, assists and encourages learning to feel, aids trust, promotes speaking out; helps to strengthen inner security and sense of safety; promotes trust in Goddess and the Light, increases trust in oneself and one's life, encourages inner peace

TIGER LILY
(Hymerocallis fuireia)
(Belly) Orange

> **Add Gemstones:** Orange Calcite, Honey Calcite, Red Jasper, Orange Sapphire, Carnelian, Carnelian Agate, Red Aventurine, Orange Zincite, Clear Quartz Crystal, Danburite

> Supports sexuality, fertility and reproduction on the emotional level; heals past sexual abuse, facilitates rape recovery; aids in reaching out to others, promotes starting new relationships after sexual trauma; supports and promotes conception and childbearing, aids in bringing a child into incarnation, helps being a responsible lover and a responsible parent

TORCH GINGER
(Alpinia purpurata)
(Perineum) Red

> **Add Gemstones:** Ruby, Red Coral, Red Spinel, Garnet, Red Pietersite, Black Tourmaline, Obsidian, Smoky Quartz, Clear Quartz Crystal, Danburite

> For joining one's spiritual and physical life forces, brings the spiritual into the physical, connects the soul to the body, makes all acts of physical life into spiritual acts; aids in manifesting one's life purpose, promotes spiritualized sexuality; encourages effort, courage, endurance, responsibility; promotes fertility, aids in healing past sexual abuse, lifts depression

TREE OF GOLD
(Tabebuia argentea)

(Solar Plexus) Yellow

> **Add Gemstones:** Yellow Opal, Golden Topaz, Yellow Sunstone, Golden Beryl, Clear Beryl, Golden Labradorite, White Moonstone, Rainbow Moonstone, Clear Quartz Crystal, Danburite
>
> Supports those in service to others and the planet, supports those on the Bodhisattva Path; helps with connecting to higher wisdom and the Light; aids those who teach to present clear ideas and to teach effectively; helps healers and others in service to prevent and heal burnout, rejuvenates and regenerates; aids in manifesting karmic gifts and rewards; helps those in service to see the positive results of their work

TREE ORCHID
(Bauhinia variegata)

(Crown) Lavender

> **Add Gemstones:** Sugilite, Pink Fluorite, Amethyst, Canadian Amethyst, Pink Tourmaline, Alexandrite, Charoite, Herkimer Diamond, Danburite
>
> Deepens meditation, encourages spiritual opening, increases all psychic abilities and assists in learning how to use them; spiritualizes daily life, spiritualizes love relationships, promotes the will to attain enlightenment in this lifetime; increases one's connection with the Light and Light Be-ings, pairs the serious student with Light Be-ing teachers--spirit guides, angels, Goddess; heals the emotional, mental and spiritual bodies; promotes unconditional love and understanding the oneness of all life

TRUMPET CREEPER
(Campsis grandiflora)
(Belly) Orange

> **Add Gemstones:** Pecos Quartz, Carnelian, Red Phantom Quartz, Peach Moonstone, Vanadinite, Orange Zincite, Red Jasper, Clear Quartz Crystal, Danburite
>
> Safely releases emotions; clears anger, heals emotional trauma, helps to heal sexual and emotional abuse, aids sexual dysfunction, releases old resentments; ends being stuck by releasing the blocks--the release may be intensive; promotes a major increase in healing and well-being after emotional release; completes old emotional business to permit moving forward and going on with one's life; promotes transformations

TRUMPET CREEPER
(Campsis radicans)
(Root) Red

> **Add Gemstones:** Garnet, Mexican Opal, Ruby, Amethyst, Amethyst with Hematite, Pecos Quartz, Moroccan Red Quartz, Herkimer Diamond, Danburite
>
> Attracts joy and brings it into one's daily life; clears and purifies the kundalini and hara lines, removes energetic obstructions to the manifesting of joy, heals sadness on the emotional and mental body levels; promotes connection with Goddess and the Light, reminds that "you are Goddess" (Goddess within), brings the Higher Self into the physical body; promotes core soul healing, offers karmic healing, repairs the DNA; helps in the ascension/enlightenment process, encourages living a joyful spiritual life

TRUMPET CREEPER
(Campsis radicans)

(Solar Plexus) Yellow

> **Add Gemstones:** Yellow Sunstone, Yellow Opal, Golden Topaz, Citrine, Yellow Fluorite, Lemon Yellow Calcite, Yellow Zincite, Clear Quartz Crystal, Danburite
>
> Cleanses, clears and purifies; promotes chakra clearing and clearing of energy channels, increases energy flows, aids running energy and bringing in Light energy; releases attachments and negative entities from the aura, offers protection from negative interference; promotes balanced psychic opening and development, aids astral travel with safe return to the body; good essence to use in a sprayer for crystal clearing

VIOLET
(Viola odorata)

(Third Eye) Blue

> **Add Gemstones:** Blue Dumortierite, Blue Aventurine, Iolite, Azurite, Blue Tourmaline, Lapis Lazuli, Blue Sapphire, Snow Quartz, Clear Quartz Crystal, Danburite
>
> Promotes spiritual growth and psychic opening, aids in choosing a spiritual path and purpose, helps one to see the sacred in the everyday, aids beginning a spiritual path; aids opening to psychic discovery, initiates clairvoyance and clairaudience, begins one's connection with Goddess and the Light; promotes integrity, encourages pleasantness in spiritual interactions with others, purifies, calms. Victorian symbol for modesty or faithfulness, also called Sweet Violet or Blue Violet.

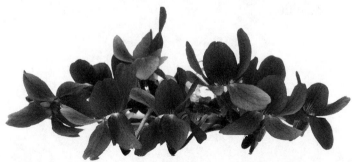

VIOLET
(Viola biflora)
(Solar Plexus) Yellow

> **Add Gemstones:** Natural Citrine, Yellow Opal, Golden Amber, Lemon Yellow Calcite, Golden Labradorite, Golden Beryl, Septarian, Herkimer Diamond, Danburite
>
> Assists early psychic opening, promotes telepathy (sending rather than receiving) of psychic images and information; initiates learning and practicing psychic healing, aids in learning to visualize; acts as a mental stimulant, enhances memorization and promotes good study habits; protects, fills the aura with Light. Victorians used this flower as a symbol of rural living, of happiness in the country. Also called Yellow Violet or Yellow Wood Violet

WAND FLOWER
(Sparaxis grandiflora)
(Heart Complex) Mixed Colors—pink, red, orange, yellow, white

> **Add Gemstones:** Rose Aura Crystal, Gem Rose Quartz, Pink Sapphire, Pink Tourmaline, Pink Kunzite, White Moonstone, Herkimer Diamond, Danburite
>
> Heals and repairs the heart chakra on all levels (heart complex); promotes joy in work and working in joy, promotes the work of one's hands reflecting the joy in one's heart, assists finding work that is what you love to do, supports doing work you love; a good essence for hands-on healers, prevents burnout, prevents boredom and loss of interest in one's true work and life path

WATER HYACINTH
(Eichbornia crassipes)

(Crown) Lavender

Add Gemstones: Charoite, Amethyst, Ametrine, Lepidolite, Sugilite, Purple Fluorite, Violet Tourmaline, Alexandrite, Herkimer Diamond, Danburite

Brings and manifests spiritual blessings, promote inner growth, promotes inner peace, increases spiritual nourishment and fulfillment; provide stronger connection with Goddess, spirit guides, angels, and other Light Be-ings; fosters the feeling of being held safe and loved in the Goddess's arms; heals insomnia and fear, prevents nightmares and night terrors; calms, promotes trust, offers a peaceful gentle death at one's time of transition

WATER LILY
(Nymphae capensis)

(Crown) Purple

Add Gemstones: Amethyst, Charoite, Lepidolite, Purple Fluorite, Sugilite, Moonstone, Angel Wing Selenite, Seraphanite, Herkimer Diamond, Danburite

Helps transcend suffering to attain spiritual wisdom, aids in becoming an old soul; aids in achieving guidance from one's soul, promotes contact with angels and spirit guides, enhances spiritual growth and evolution; supports spiritual transformation on all levels, helps in attaining enlightenment in this lifetime; aids in fulfilling karmic obligations and healing karmic patterns

WATER LILY
(Nymphae caerulea)
(Third Eye) Blue

> **Add Gemstones:** Lapis Lazuli, Blue Aventurine, Azurite, Sodalite, Celestite, Blue Kunzite, Blue Sapphire, Iolite, Blue Labradorite, Herkimer Diamond, Danburite
>
> Increases one's ability to receive the wisdom of the ancients, accesses star wisdom, accesses wisdom from other galaxies and planets; promotes and increases the range of channeling and other psychic abilities (clairvoyance, clairaudience, crystal gazing, telepathy, empathy, psychic knowing, etc.); opens and strengthens psychic potential, cleanses and heals the energy bodies; provides connection through the Earth grid with the angelic realm, aids ability to contact and learn from Ascended Masters and the Lords of Karma; an all-healing plant and essence

WATER LILY
(Nymphae Denver)
(Throat) White

> **Add Gemstones:** Blue Andean Opal, Amazonite, Turquoise, Gem Silica, Blue Calcite, Blue Aventurine, Angelite, Blue Apophyllite, Celestite, Herkimer Diamond, Danburite
>
> Good essence for Earth healers; stimulates Earth awareness and awareness of planetary stewardship; promotes honoring the oneness of all life, inspires compassion for all that lives; increases empathy, assists in receiving psychic information from devas, elementals, water spirits, Earth spirits, whales and dolphins; helps those who participate in Earth change healing for themselves, others and the planet; supports incarnated bodhisattvas; aids all psychic abilities, heals burnout in psychics and healers

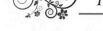

WATER LILY
(Nymphae virginalis)
(Transpersonal Point) White

> **Add Gemstones:** White Opal, Selenite, White Moonstone, Clear Beryl, White Apophyllite, White Topaz, Snow Quartz, Phenacite, Clear Quartz Crystal, Danburite

> Cleanses and clears all the bodies and aura levels, opens and aligns the bodies, clears chakra obstructions and blocks, clears obstructions from the energy channels at all levels; removes negative attachments and entities, releases past life artifacts, aids karmic clearing and release, heals negativity; fills the aura, chakras, bodies and channels with Light, brings in information and healing; increases one's connection and conscious contact with Goddess; regenerates, repairs and heals

WHITE FLAG
(Spathyphyllum sp.)
(Third Eye) White

> **Add Gemstones:** Snow Quartz, White Phantom Quartz, Moonstone, Green Aventurine, Green Jade, Serpentine Jade, Emerald, Green Jasper, Clear Quartz Crystal, Danburite

> Offers protection for those who are shy or vulnerable; provides comfort in social situations, aids self-confidence and positive assertiveness, promotes emotional and spiritual growth, promotes growth of social skills; increases ability to reach out to others, helps those who feel unwanted; good essence for adolescents and those who have too often been told to be silent

WILLOW, Pussy
(Salix discolor)
(Vision) Grey

> **Add Gemstones:** Clear Fluorite, Phenacite, Aragonite, Phantom Quartz, Labradorite, Inclusion Quartz, Grey Moonstone, Silver Aura Crystal, Herkimer Diamond, Danburite

> Increases psychic vision and enhances understanding of psychic information from all the senses; stimulates the viewing of past lives and past life situations that need understanding and release; promotes psychic healing, increases range of telepathy (sending rather than receiving of psychic messages and energy); repairs the psychic sensory channels and chakras, repairs the causal and galactic bodies (higher level energy bodies) of this-life and past life injury, heals core soul damage; causes strong psychic opening that may be intense

WISTERIA
(Wisterian sinensis)
(Third Eye) Blue

> **Add Gemstones:** Avalonite, Azurite, Blue Chalcedony, Lapis Lazuli, Blue Aventurine, Angelite, Blue Sapphire, Iolite, Clear Quartz Crystal, Danburite

> Aids the ability to communicate with highest level Light Beings--angelic presences, spirit guides, otherplanetary healers and helpers, one's soul, and the Goddess; aids psychic opening, strengthens psychic healing and self-healing, promotes clairvoyance, clairaudience and channeling; inspires becoming a channel for the highest level psychic healing and information; promotes spiritual evolution and enlightenment

YARROW
(Achillea millefolium)

(Solar Plexus) Multi Colors—White, Pink, Yellow

Add Gemstones: Fresh Water Pearl, Amber, Lepidolite with Mica, Selenite, Golden Selenite, Rose Quartz, Dravite, Citrine, Clear Quartz Crystal, Danburite

Shields the kundalini chakras from negativity and psychic draining (psychic vampirism); protects and clears healers who take in the pain of others and feel it in themselves; heals burnout, exhaustion, fatigue, vulnerability and stress especially in healers; buffers and protects, cleanses and clears, heals and supports; good essence for healers, social workers, activists, planet healers, and all who do service work

YARROW
(Achillea millefolium)

(Heart) Pink

Add Gemstones: Pink Kunzite, Pink Tourmaline, Morganite, Pink Chinese Opal, Mangano Calcite, Pink Calcite, Clear Quartz Crystal, Danburite

Heals and protects the vulnerable heart, promotes this life and past life emotional healing, releases heart scars gently, heals emotional trauma, aids emotional body healing, heals heartache and betrayal, soothes grief; brings a sense of safety, security and joy; promotes peace, love and trust, allows unconditional love to begin, provides emotional protection

YARROW
(Achillea millefolium)
(Perineum) Red

Add Gemstones: Cuprite, Red Phantom Quartz, Ruby, Star Ruby, Pecos Quartz, Moroccan Red Quartz, Red Coral, Hematite, Clear Quartz Crystal, Danburite

Heals the life force and the energy bodies' ability to bring in and assimilate life force energy; heals damage occurred during incarnating, repairs damage to the life force channels from this and other lifetimes, heals the karma of incarnational damage; offers karmic healing and karmic grace, promotes core soul healing; heals and inspires the will to live, increases passion for living, inspires love of life, stimulates sexual passion

YARROW
(Achillea millefolium)
(Transpersonal Point) White

Add Gemstones: White Moonstone, White Fresh Water Pearl, Snow Quartz, Phenacite, White Sapphire, Clear Beryl, Clear Kunzite, Herkimer Diamond, Danburite

Promotes spiritual purity and aids and protects those who are pure of spirit, offers spiritual protection and protection of innocence; all-aura clearing and cleansing, releases and removes negative entities, attachments, possessions; ends negative interference and repairs damage from psychic attacks; heals the aura of rips, tears, holes and other damage; promotes increased psychic and spiritual evolution with full protection; fills the aura with Light, purity, beauty and love

YARROW
(Achillea sp.)

(Solar Plexus) Yellow

Add Gemstones: Natural Citrine, Pyrite, Golden Topaz, Golden Beryl, Golden Labradorite, Yellow Sunstone, Tiger Eye, Clear Quartz Crystal, Danburite

Provides protection from negative interference and negative energies; repels and releases psychic attacks, removes and destroys negative entities, ends vulnerability to possession; protects from other peoples' jealousy, envy and malice; shields from others' negative thoughts and emotions; prevents psychic vampires (grasping needy people) from hooking on; promotes a positive outlook and steadiness under stress and attack; protects the curious from harm, increases courage, raises mood

YESTERDAY TODAY AND TOMORROW
(Brunfelcia)

(Third Eye) Blue

Add Gemstones: Cobalt Aura Crystal, Angelite, Azurite, Blue Aventurine, Lapis Lazuli, Sodalite, Blue Sapphire, Celestite, Blue Quartz, Clear uartz Crystal, Danburite

Breaks the bonds of the negative past, heals emotional and mental attachments and harmful karmic patterns; promotes letting go of old traumas, wounds, hurts and resentments; promotes karmic breakthroughs and healing of past lives; heals from the higher body levels for more complete core soul healing; aids connection, communication and guidance from angels, spirit guides, protectors and the Lords of Karma; promotes breakthroughs and transformations that heal on all levels

ZEPHYR LILY
(Zephyranthes grandiflora)
(Crown) Lavender

Add Gemstones: Selenite, Purple Kunzite, Rutile Amethyst, Pink Calcite, Violet Tourmaline, Sugilite, Pink Sapphire, Herkimer Diamond, Danburite

For lasting bliss and eternal peace, provides rest from jobs well done, heals burnout and exhaustion; offers love, peace, wellness, well-being, joy; promotes full spiritual awareness of the Goddess and Goddess within, inspires full awareness of everlasting love and unconditional love, gives full understanding of the oneness of all life; supports enlightenment (ascension) and all spiritual processes and practices; provides understanding of one's place in the universe, offers inner peace and the certainty of being loved

Healing with Flower and Gemstone Essences

by Diane Stein
ISBN: 978-0-9406-7699-2
160 pp pb • $10.95

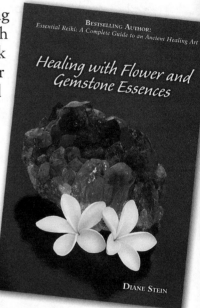

A comprehensive modern guide to making and using flower essences at home, with flowers from your own garden. The book describes how to make and use over 200 of Diane Stein's unique flower and gemstone essence combinations.

The flowers and gemstones are described in detail, with information on the kundalini and hara line chakras and how to match essences to them. Contains an extensive dictionary of everyday flowers--and the optional gemstones to use with them and enhance them--for every healing need.

Diane Stein shows you how to:

- Make and use flower essences
- Use the kundalini chakras and the hara line
- Use flowers from your own garden

Available at bookstores and natural food stores nationwide or order your copy directly by sending cost of item plus $2.50 shipping/handling ($.75 s/h for each additional copy ordered at the same time) to:

Lotus Press, PO Box 325, Twin Lakes, WI 53181 USA
toll free order line: 800 824 6396 • office phone: 262 889 856 • office fax: 262 889 2461
email: lotuspress@lotuspress.com • web site: www.lotuspress.com

Lotus Press is the publisher of a wide range of books and software in the field of alternative health, including Ayurveda, Chinese medicine, herbology, aromatherapy, Reiki and energetic healing modalities. Request our free book catalog.